"THE POLIO PARADOX is heaven sent.
Thank you, Dr. Bruno, for writing a book for US!"
—KATHY GALLETLY, EDITOR, *Independent Polio News*

"Wow! I have spina bifida and I read
THE POLIO PARADOX from beginning to end.
What an eye-opener for *anyone* with a disability. . . .Thanks
to Dr. Bruno for leading me on the next chapter of
my life . . . the one where I stop doing for everyone else
and start caring for and taking care of myself."
—VICKI BRASEL

"Explains exactly what damage was done by
the polio virus and how that damage is causing
our present symptoms. Thank you, Dr. Bruno, for
showing us the way to a better, more satisfying life."
—BETH TURNER, R.N.

"A must read for everyone . . .
get THE POLIO PARADOX for yourself. Then get
an extra copy for your family and be sure to get a third
copy for your doctor. . . .You will be amazed and uplifted."
—DIANNE DE PAUL, BOARD MEMBER, POLIO SURVIVORS PLUS

ALSO BY RICHARD L. BRUNO:

How to STOP Being Vampire Bait:
The Stress Annihilation Workbook

The Post-Polio Sequelae Monograph Series

The Post-Polio Workbook

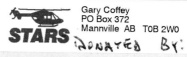
PRAISE FOR *THE POLIO PARADOX*

"The similarities between CFS and PPS
are tantalizing. Dr. Bruno's work is immensely
important to those with CFS and PPS."
—DR. DAVID BELL, CHRONIC FATIGUE SYNDROME SPECIALIST

"Dr. Bruno's uncanny humor and wit make the book
read like a story. . . .Gives you a plan on how to get
your life back . . . a must for all polio survivors."
—JENNY DANIELSON, PRESIDENT,
TRIAD POST-POLIO SUPPORT GROUP

"Dr. Bruno has provided practical strategies to minimize
the secondary effects of disability and maximize quality
of life. With [this book], he emphasizes that
these strategies are equally beneficial to those of us
with cerebral palsy, spina bifida, and a variety of
other long-term disabilities. Thank you, Dr. Bruno!"
—DR. BONNIE MOULTON, TEMPLE UNIVERSITY

"I cannot stop reading this book! I've never been so excited
reading about PPS. It is amazing, Dr. Bruno's talent to put
across what polio survivors need to know in understandable
language. THE POLIO PARADOX is absolutely fantastic.
I recommend it to the whole world!"
—CILLA WEBSTER, PRESIDENT, POST-POLIO NETWORK SA

"A must read . . . addresses the physiological and,
maybe more important, the psychological aspects of
the late effects of poliomyelitis . . . makes it possible
for professionals and polio survivors alike to grasp
the physical and the psychological complexities of PPS."
—NICKIE LANCASTER, R.N., COORDINATOR,
POLIO HEROES OF TENNESSEE

 more . . .

"Marvelous . . . groundbreaking . . . a wiring diagram
and operator's manual for the chronically fatiqued
body and brain. . . . Dr. Bruno's treatment program for
chronic fatigue has amply proved its worth."
—DR. ELIZABETH DOWSETT, FOUNDER,
CFS DIAGNOSTIC AND MANAGEMENT SERVICE

"I am an R.N. with Post-Polio Syndrome. . . . Dr. Bruno
helps with the choices we must make to continue to
be independent, and he does it in a gentle yet persuasive
manner. Read THE POLIO PARADOX.
It might save your life!"
—PATRICIA CUDAHY, R.N.

"Outstanding . . . remarkable . . . tells the truth
about PPS and in so doing frees us polio survivors
to move from disabled to enabled. . . .The author's warmth
and compassion shine throughout the book. . . .
With great clarity, Bruno dispels the confusion
surrounding this sequel to polio."
—VICKI MCKENNA, AUTHOR OF *A Balanced Way of Living:
Practical and Holistic Strategies for Coping with PPS*

"*Finally* someone who knows has written a book about
Post-Polio Sequelae! THE POLIO PARADOX is the
first book about and for polio survivors and the
medical community. . . . Dr. Bruno reveals that we
can learn to live within our NEW abilities."
—CAROLEANNE GREEN, DIRECTOR,
NATIONAL POLIO CARE ASSOCIATES

THE
POLIO
PARADOX

UNDERSTANDING AND TREATING
"POST-POLIO SYNDROME"
AND CHRONIC FATIGUE

RICHARD L. BRUNO, H.D., PH.D.

WARNER BOOKS

An AOL Time Warner Company

To the world's twenty million polio survivors,
especially our patients and research participants;

To Maureen Egen,
who made *The Polio Paradox* possible;

To Nancy,
who makes all things possible.

PUBLISHER'S NOTE: This book is not intended as a substitute for medical advice of physicians. The reader should regularly consult a physician in all matters relating to his or her health, and particularly in respect of any symptoms that may require diagnosis or medical attention.

Grateful acknowledgment is given for permission to use the photo of Joanne Kelly on the cover, the poem "Where Is That Little Girl?" by Ruth Mihalenko on page 92, and the artwork by Alice Rumpler on page 225.

Warner Books, Inc., 1271 Avenue of the Americas, New York, NY 10020
Visit our Web site at www.twbookmark.com.

An AOL Time Warner Company

Printed in the United States of America
Originally published in hardcover by Warner Books, Inc.
First Trade Printing: June 2003
10 9 8 7 6 5 4 3 2 1

Hardcover ISBN: 0-446-52907-9
Paperback ISBN: 0-446-69069-4
Library of Congress Control Number: 2002103347

OF SPECIAL INTEREST TO THOSE WITH:

Myalgic Encephalomyelitis
Chronic Fatigue Syndrome
Guillain-Barre Syndrome
Transverse Myelitis
Gulf War Syndrome
Chronic Headaches
Multiple Sclerosis
Chronic Back Pain
Spinal Cord Injury
West Nile Virus
Cerebral Palsy
Fibromyalgia
Spina Bifida

ACKNOWLEDGMENTS

With gratitude and profound appreciation to:

All of the polio survivors who have contributed their personal stories, especially Sir Arthur C. Clarke; His Eminence, The Most Reverend Edward Cardinal Egen; The Honorable Fred Grandy; and Lt. Governor John Hagar;

Kate Anderson for her generosity, eagle eye, continuous creativity, and wicked wit;

Burt Bacharach for "scoring" the past thirty-three years;

Geri Barry and the George A. Ohl, Jr., Infantile Paralysis Foundation for continuous support and her rapid response under very difficult circumstances;

Laura Belder for everything, especially keeping the S.S. PPI steaming ahead;

Eleanor Bodian for her most helpful history lessons;

Barry Corbet for giving a new writer his first chance and always making the words better;

Ray Coulton of "Co-Cure" and Chris Salter of Lincolnshire Polio Network for keeping me effortlessly up to date;

Dr. Elizabeth Dowsett and Lydia Nelson of the National ME/FM Action Network for their support of our work and making the 2001 International Chronic Fatigue Survey possible;

Brandan Falsey and my luncheon companions, the citizens of the Boro of Arrowhead County;

Mia and Thaddeus Farrow and Chris Templeton for unselfishly giving of themselves to the Post-Polio Letter campaign;

Alan Fiore at Mada Design for his collaboration and remarkable illustrations;

Dr. Nancy Frick, whose insights and contributions are to be found on nearly every page;

Dr. Ray Goetz for "admitting" me to P.I.

Carolyn Lamontagne Hall and Tae Won Kim for volunteering their time and computer expertise;

Janis Hirsh and Tom Fontana for opening the swinging door to "Elsewhere";

Jackie Joiner for her most constructive criticism and walking me through the wonderful world of Time Warner;

Daniel Kane, the staff and the administration of Englewood Hospital and Medical Center for their unstinting support of The Post-Polio Institute and The International Centre for Post-Polio Education and Research;

Kathy Linder and Lea Sabaugh for responding to almost daily harassment with an avalanche of articles and much good humor;

Mary—and especially Mary—for keeping us well stocked and well cared for;

Kathy McCullough for her unflagging spirit, willingness to be such a good "bad" cop, and her efforts heeding—and going above and beyond—the call of duty;

Maureen McGovern and her Works of Heart Foundation for collaborating to develop a music therapy program to treat stress in polio survivors;

Leslie Moonves and CBS for helping to inform North America about PPS;

David Morse for being the first to give of himself — and to continuing giving — to help polio survivors;

Natalie's of Ridgewood for nourishing body and heart;

Dr. Joe Nuziale (and Grace) for keeping me straight;

The Pilgrim Sands for revitalizing mind and soul;

The Post-Polio Institute team for their compassion, competence, and the joy of working together;

Sugar Rautbord for broadening the scope of this book;

Debra Refson for being "The Nexus," for her motivating logic, remarkable insights, and the idea for distributing The Post-Polio Letter;

Gerard Shorb, David Bodian Collection archivist, the Alan Mason Chesney Archives of the Johns Hopkins Medical Institutions; and Maggie Yax, Albert B. Sabin archivist, Cincinnati Medical Heritage Center, University of Cincinnati Medical Center;

Springfield College, where my life began and the seeds were planted;

Dr. Jerry Zimmerman for a friendship and collaboration spanning a millennium;

In Memoriam: Audrey, Carl, David, John, Judi, Ken, Margaret, Niccola and Robert, Reverend Ken Childs, Russ Berrie and Dr. David Bodian.

CONTENTS

par•a•dox (par' e-doks') n.
From the Greek: Conflicting with expectation.
1. A seemingly contradictory statement that may nonethe-less be true.
2. One exhibiting inexplicable or contradictory aspects.
3. An assertion that is essentially self-contradictory, though based on a valid deduction from acceptable premises.
4. A statement contrary to received opinion.

American Heritage Dictionary

Patty slowly limped into my office, leaning heavily on a walker. Her husband followed behind, also seeming to limp, weighed down by shopping bags filled with years of medical records and pounds of X rays. Patty collapsed into a chair. Small and slender, she looked much younger than her fifty-eight years. Black hair framed a pale face showing fatigue, pain, fear, and anger. She fixed me with dark eyes that filled with tears as she said, "I don't want surgery, again!"

I handed Patty tissues and, as she cried, I began looking through her ream of medical reports. During two long years she had had the proverbial "million-dollar workup." Her family doctor started with the standard blood tests and chest X ray, even a virus culture and test for Lyme disease. When all results came back negative, Patty was shipped off to local specialists, where the exotic testing began. The new test battery read like a Wall Street ticker: ANA, ACE, ANCA(C), ANCA(P), MMA, PE, RPR, SPEP. When these results, too, revealed no physical illness, Patty was asked the inevitable question: "Do you think you're depressed?"

"Of course I'm depressed," she told the doctors. "I'm exhausted all the time. I can't stay awake during the day, but I can't sleep at night. I have trouble swallowing. My legs burn and aren't strong enough to take me from one end of the house to the other. And my low back always hurts."

Ah! Low back pain. Now that was something the doctors could deal with. So Patty began a new round of studies with a new batch of specialists. She had CAT scans of the chest, abdomen, and pelvis. Somatosensory evoked potentials. MRIs of the brain, neck, and upper back—and, eureka, they found something! Patty had a herniated disc in her neck. Excited by finally finding something abnormal, the doctors sent Patty to the most prestigious university teaching hospital in Manhattan. There she underwent painful studies reminiscent of tests performed on her when she'd had polio. She had a spinal tap, a myelogram in which dye was injected into her spinal fluid, and another MRI, this time with dye injected into her blood. These tests confirmed that she had a herniated disc in her neck but did not explain her exhaustion, her trouble sleeping, swallowing, and walking, or even her low back pain. Yet the neurologist recommended another MRI and a consultation with a neurosurgeon to discuss removing the herniated disc, despite the fact that his report stated he could not blame any of her symptoms on that disc.

Not one of nearly a dozen doctors took into account the simple fact that Patty had had polio. "I told them all," she said. And sure enough, in each and every doctor's report was the same sentence: "History of childhood polio." Even if Patty hadn't told them about the polio, it was obvious. Just by watching her walk it was clear that her left leg was much shorter, smaller, and weaker than her right. I asked how her odyssey of doctor visits and medical tests had begun. Patty sighed and said, "I told the doctor my legs felt weak."

Leg weakness and burning muscles. Exhaustion. Trouble sleeping and swallowing. And, of course, back pain. How many polio survivors like Patty have I seen during the past twenty years? How many patients have come to The Post-Polio Institute after having the million-dollar workup that found "no medical cause" for their symptoms? How many polio survivors around the world have been turned away by doctor after doctor, being told that their symptoms were the result of depression or all in their heads? The answer is tens of thousands.

When I met Patty I couldn't help but shake my head and wonder what year it was. Was it 1978, when no one in the medical community knew that polio survivors were having new symptoms: overwhelming fatigue, muscle weakness, muscle and joint pain, sleep disorders, heightened sensitivity to anesthesia, cold and pain, and difficulty swallowing and breathing? Was it 1984, before an article in *Newsweek* announced to America that polio survivors were experiencing "The Late Effects of Polio"? Was it 1991, before every orthopedist and rehabilitation medicine specialist in the country had received three special issues of the journal *Orthopedics* devoted to something called "post-polio sequelae"? Was it even 1995, before the New York Academy of Sciences published the proceedings of an international symposium on "post-polio syndrome"?

No, I met Patty in 2001, twenty years after hundreds of thousands of polio survivors had made clear, and more than fifteen years after the American medical establishment and even the federal government had accepted, that something was indeed wrong inside the bodies of those who survived polio more than forty years before. How could Patty's doctors not know this? How could they have treated—and not treated—her this way?

Patty's experience made me realize that she and all polio survivors are caught in a paradox:

POLIO WAS THOUGHT TO BE A "STABLE DISEASE." ONCE POLIO SURVIVORS RECOVERED MUSCLE STRENGTH AFTER THE POLIO ATTACK, THEIR PHYSICAL ABILITIES WERE SUPPOSED TO REMAIN FOR THE REST OF THEIR LIVES. HOWEVER, CONTRARY TO THIS COMMON BELIEF, POLIO SURVIVORS' STRENGTH AND ABILITIES WERE EBBING AWAY.

Patty's exasperating, exhausting, and hurtful experiences with her doctors revealed a second painful paradox:

IN THE 1980S, DOCTORS WERE IGNORING AND REJECTING THE SAME POLIO SURVIVORS WHOSE PLIGHT HAD RIVETED THE ATTENTION OF THE WORLD'S MEDICAL COMMUNITY AND SPURRED IT TO ACTION JUST THIRTY YEARS BEFORE.

It's unacceptable that in the year 2002 polio survivors like Patty are being forced to run such expensive, painful, and unproductive medical gauntlets. With twenty years of articles describing "The Late Effects of Polio," published in journals that include the *Journal of the American Medical Association* and *New England Journal of Medicine,* doctors have no excuse for treating polio survivors' new and disabling symptoms as indications of mental illness or rejecting them as a matter of faith, something in which doctors choose not to believe. With volumes of information now available on the Internet with a point and a click, no polio survivor should be told that overwhelming fatigue is "just a symptom of depression," that muscle weakness is "all in your head," or that the late effects of polio "do not exist."

There is no question that polio survivors' new symptoms are real—and that there's no more time to waste in treating them. Half of North America's estimated 1.8 million polio survivors are in their forties, fifties, and sixties, at the peak of their careers, the apogee of their lives, and they are watching as new symptoms cause their ability to work and function ebb away. This need not happen! After two decades of research, we know why polio survivors are having new problems, and we know how to treat and manage them. It is time to set forth the facts—to set the record straight—once and for all.

PART ONE

In the Beginning . . .

CHAPTER 1

In the Beginning

One winter morning I happened to take a phone call in my office at Columbia-Presbyterian Medical Center from a thirty-six-year-old polio survivor from New Jersey. He told me he had developed weakness in one arm and had been given a death sentence. Weakness on one side of the body is a symptom of amyotrophic lateral sclerosis—ALS or Lou Gehrig's disease—the progressive and fatal neurological disease that took the life of Morrie in *Tuesdays with Morrie*. The neurologist who examined him said, because of the weakness in his one arm, that he must have "some kind of ALS" and that there was nothing to be done. This polio survivor from New Jersey was calling to ask if I'd done any research that would tell him how long he had to live.

But something was very wrong.

"You had one arm completely paralyzed by polio as a child?" I asked.

"Yes," he said.

"And the other arm that's been doing all the work for your paralyzed arm is now weak."

"Yes."

"You only have one arm that could become weak."

"Yes," he said with a sigh.

I told him I'd call back and went to Robert Darling, the

chairman emeritus of the Department of Rehabilitation Medicine at Columbia University's College of Physicians and Surgeons. I asked what happens to polio survivors when they get older. "They get weaker and tired," he said.

I called the man from New Jersey and asked him to come to Columbia-Presbyterian, where testing quickly revealed that he did not have ALS, that he was not going to die. But his arm was indeed weak. The question was why?

It's hard to believe that this phone call came twenty years ago. I had just finished my doctorate and was training as a fellow in the Department of Rehabilitation Medicine at Columbia University's College of Physicians and Surgeons. I was studying and treating patients with disorders of the autonomic nervous system, the "automatic" nervous system that regulates blood flow, blood pressure, heart rate, and sweating. When that New Jersey polio survivor called, I was studying an enigmatic and searingly painful condition called causalgia. We were discovering that the autonomic nervous system in patients with causalgia was unable to regulate the amount of blood flowing to their hands and feet.

What caught my attention as much as the gentleman's increasing weakness was that his polio-affected arm had always been colder than his "good" arm. Indeed, his skin on the "polio side" was cold to the touch, suggesting that something was wrong with blood flow to the arm. Since I was already studying problems with blood flow, I naturally wanted to find out what was happening to his. And I also wondered if other polio survivors were having similar problems. So I called New York and New Jersey disability organizations to find subjects to come to Columbia in 1983 and participate in our first laboratory study, which looked at the effects of temperature on polio survivors.

And polio survivors did come, as willing research subjects and for help. The more survivors I met, the more problems I heard about and the more questions needed answers. In addition to muscle weakness and cold skin, polio survivors were reporting physical and mental fatigue, joint and muscle pain, even difficulty breathing and swallowing. These reports prompted the first of our five questionnaire surveys of more than 2500 polio survivors to find out about their polio and post-polio experiences, the symptoms they are having and what triggers them, and how they feel emotionally about their experiences and symptoms.

From Nothing to *Nightline*

Since Columbia-Presbyterian is in New York City, the media started to get wind of our research. In April 1984 *Newsweek* published the first national magazine article about polio survivors' new problems, which described our work and featured polio survivor and post-polio researcher Nancy Frick, whom you will meet in chapter 15. In May I presented our findings on the effects of cold at the first international research symposium on the late effects of polio, which was attended by only thirty-two doctors. At the conference I agreed to organize a task force that would work to promote communication among interested doctors and researchers, educate the medical community and polio survivors about the new symptoms, identify funding for research, and promote the acceptance of the late effects of polio as a medical diagnosis for which government benefits should be provided.

By 1985 the story of the late effects of polio, now dubbed a medical mystery, was sweeping the country. Developer of the oral polio vaccine Albert Sabin and I appeared on ABC's *Nightline,* the first national television broadcast about polio survivors' new problems. Later that year members of the newly formed Post-Polio Research Task Force wrote the guidelines that would allow polio survivors who could no longer work to receive Social Security disability benefits. The publishers of the journal *Orthopedics* asked me to edit a special issue on the late effects of polio, which had been renamed post-polio sequelae—the "sequel" to polio. This issue was mailed free of charge to every orthopedist and rehabilitation medicine specialist in the United States.

By 1987 the depth and breadth of polio survivors' problems were undeniable. That year the Public Health Service's National

Health Interview Survey estimated that there were 1.63 million polio survivors alive in the United States, many more than anyone had ever imagined. There were more polio survivors than those with Parkinson's disease, multiple sclerosis, and spinal cord injury combined. The same survey found that nearly 60 percent of paralytic and 30 percent of nonparalytic polio survivors were having new symptoms and losing their ability to function. What made these findings all the more disturbing was that neither polio survivors nor doctors realized that these problems were occurring and that polio survivors were not receiving medical care or government benefits to help them if they could no longer work. With every new polio survivor we met, it became more and more clear that much needed to be done if polio survivors were going to get the help they needed and deserved.

To introduce PPS to a national scientific audience, in 1986 I organized and moderated a symposium at the annual meeting of the American Association for the Advancement of Science. Also that year, I asked actor David Morse to help get the facts out about PPS by filming a public service announcement on the set of *St. Elsewhere,* and he readily agreed. In 1987, when David and I went to Washington, D.C., to unveil the announcement, we found ourselves on an even more important mission. The guidelines for polio survivors' Social Security disability benefits that Task Force members had written in 1985 had been shelved in favor of benefits for those with AIDS. Disability benefits should not be an either–or proposition, which is the message David and I brought to Capitol Hill. We met with several Senate staffers who heard our case. But it was only Senator Bill Bradley who met with us in person and then wrote a letter to the Social Security commissioner asking that polio survivors receive the disability benefits to which they were entitled. On August 8, 1987, I received a letter saying that polio survivors would be allowed to receive federal disability income and that benefits guidelines were being released—guidelines that are even now being revised and expanded thanks to the efforts of New Jersey congressman Steve Rothman.

By 1988 our research and our clinical experience since 1982

had made it clear that there were not only physical but also psychological factors triggering PPS and preventing polio survivors from making the changes in their lives that were necessary to treat PPS. It appeared that our patients shared characteristics of a personality type that had been described among those who developed heart disease: the hard-driving, time-conscious, driven, self-denying, perfectionistic, overachieving "Type A" personality. We included a Type A questionnaire in the 1985 North American Survey of 676 polio survivors, who we discovered reported 50 percent more Type A behavior on average than did nondisabled individuals in the general population. What's more, the more Type A the polio survivors were, the more PPS symptoms they had, and the more severe those symptoms were.

Since the cause and treatment of PPS involved both body and mind, it was clear that polio survivors needed comprehensive treatment by a team of specialists under one roof to help them deal both physically and emotionally with the unexpected and frightening changes in their bodies. And here was yet another twist of fate. Both my undergraduate and doctoral training had been in psychophysiology, the specialty dealing with the relationship between mind and body. Psychophysiologists use the techniques of behavior modification, psychotherapy, and biofeedback to help patients feel better both physically and emotionally. These techniques were ideally suited to the minds and bodies of Type A polio survivors with PPS.

Over the River

So in 1988 I moved from Columbia to New Jersey and created the Post-Polio Rehabilitation and Research Service, whose mandate was to study the causes of PPS and apply our research findings to treat polio survivors. I assembled a team with Jerald Zimmerman, a physiatrist—a specialist in rehabilitation medicine—that included occupational, physical, and speech therapists, dietitians . . . and one psychophysiologist. Over the next ten years the team's ability to treat more and more polio survivors and to do both clinical and laboratory research expanded almost exponentially, thanks to a dozen research grants.

By 1998 the need for additional resources for our research and to treat even more polio survivors sparked the creation of The Post-Polio Institute, which allowed us to double the number of patients we could treat. We also created the Intercontinental Assessment Service, which permits us to evaluate and manage PPS in polio survivors who live far from The Institute—people from across North America and from as far away as Europe, the Middle East, South Africa, South America, Korea, and China. At The Post-Polio Institute every physical and emotional aspect of polio survivors' lives is addressed to treat and manage PPS, including obtaining assistive devices, getting wheelchair-accessible vans, making home and job modifications, and, if need be, applying for disability.

As we learned more about polio survivors and their new problems, we realized how much we didn't know. The number of questions I wanted to answer about polio survivors and PPS grew and grew. Since our first North American survey, we have conducted four International Post-Polio Surveys, in all studying nearly three thousand polio survivors and individuals without disabilities. Our Surveys have asked questions ranging from what polio survivors eat for breakfast to the symptoms associated with post-polio "brain fatigue," the frightening and sometimes dangerous effects of anesthesia, and the physical, emotional, and sexual abuse polio survivors experienced when they had polio. The Surveys, our laboratory research, and clinical studies of our patients have produced just over three dozen scientific articles and book chapters, more than two dozen articles about PPS for polio survivors in disability-related magazines, as well as a dozen books and monographs.

The facts about PPS have been getting out in other ways. In 1991 I edited two more special PPS issues of *Orthopedics*. In 1993 I gave the John Stanley Coulter Memorial Lecture to the American Congress of Rehabilitation Medicine, describing the polio experience, the needs of polio survivors, and the cause and treatment of PPS. I have been lecturing about PPS at university medical schools, hospitals, and scientific conferences, as well as to polio survivors around the world. I also advise post-polio support groups in North America, Europe, and Asia, and write the "Post-Polio Forum," a monthly column about PPS appearing in *New Mobility* magazine and on its Web site. And, maybe most importantly, every morning at seven I answer polio survivors' e-mail from around the globe.

Unfortunately, as Patty's disturbing experience illustrates, too many doctors and polio survivors still don't know about PPS. To redouble our efforts to educate polio survivors and medical professionals around the world, in 2001 I asked for a George Ohl, Jr., Infantile Paralysis Foundation grant to create The International Centre for Post-Polio Education and Research. This Centre is the new home of what's now the International Post-Polio Task Force, whose clinician, scientist, and polio survivor members in twenty-three countries on four continents distribute the latest information about the cause and treatment of PPS, help create polio clinics and support groups, and lobby governments to accept PPS as a medical diagnosis and to provide medical and disability benefits to the world's twenty million polio survivors. Also in 2001, to put all that's known about PPS in one place, to get the facts out in a clear and straightforward fashion every polio survivor can understand, I wrote *The Polio Paradox*. I've been spurred on by The International Post-Polio Task Force's motto "Every child vaccinated. Every polio survivor—and doctor—educated."

The Most Pernicious Paradox

In her autobiography, Mia Farrow (Polio Class of '54) sums up her reaction to her experience of polio at age nine:

> I saw how fragile our life structure is and how easily you can be plucked from it, and thrown into the land of uncertainty, fear, pain, and death. If polio marked the end of my childhood, it also left me with embryonic survival skills. If

you have . . . a little courage, and imagination, then you
have the internal resources to build a new life, and maybe
even a better one.

In September of last year Mia told me that she had intentionally discarded every letter, every article, every e-mail she had
received about PPS, saying, "I feel battle-weary. I don't want to
know." Could Mia have lost touch with the polio-taught survival
skills and internal resources she herself described when confronted with the possibility of PPS? If she had, she would be in
good company, since so many polio survivors are caught in the
jaws of this most pernicious Polio Paradox:

**POLIO SURVIVORS CHEATED DEATH, CONQUERED DISABILITY,
AND DEALT WITH YEARS OF SEVERE PHYSICAL AND EMO-
TIONAL PAIN TO BECOME "THE BEST AND THE BRIGHTEST,"
NOT JUST SURVIVING POLIO BUT THRIVING AND CREATING
EXTRAORDINARY PERSONAL AND PROFESSIONAL LIVES.**

**YET POLIO SURVIVORS BELIEVE THAT THEY HAVE NO SUR-
VIVAL SKILLS AT ALL, NO COURAGE, IMAGINATION, OR
INTERNAL RESOURCES TO BUILD A NEW LIFE—LET ALONE A
BETTER ONE—AND TO SURVIVE AND THRIVE WITH PPS.**

On that morning Mia confronted this Polio Paradox and found
that she had not lost touch with the truth she realized when she
was nine years old; that *all* who had polio are survivors, having
already proven that they possess the courage, imagination, and
internal resources to build a new life—and a better one—to survive and thrive with PPS. Mia agreed to start reading about the
cause, treatment, and management of PPS and to come for an
evaluation, saying "If I could survive the limbo of illness, the loss
of security, and the pain of polio, I can survive anything."

So come along on our twenty-year journey and learn the facts
about PPS. You will read about the awesome power of the
poliovirus, the damage it did inside your body—both obvious and
hidden—and the physical and psychological toll taken in those

who contracted "The Dread Disease." You will learn how damage the poliovirus did to your body so many years ago set the stage for new symptoms, and will understand what's triggering PPS today. I will describe in detail The Post-Polio Institute's program, which not only helps polio survivors stop the progression of fatigue, muscle weakness, and pain, but also allows them to decrease their symptoms and increase their ability to function—and their quality of life.

We'll also look in detail at the greatest obstacle and most difficult challenge in dealing with PPS: the psychological scars left by the polio experience. Our patients will tell you how they are terrified at the thought of an examination by a doctor or even being inside a hospital once again. You will discover that these fears cause nearly 20 percent of those who come to The Post-Polio Institute to refuse any treatment for their new symptoms. Our patients will describe the fear, anxiety, and guilt that almost invariably hinders them from making the lifestyle changes necessary to manage their new symptoms. You will learn what is required psychologically to move beyond denial and to stare down the fear and emotional pain that go along with vivid memories of the abuse and rejection that accompanied polio. You'll see how our patients are able to discard the old "use it or lose it" philosophy and learn to "conserve to preserve," accept assistive devices discarded long ago, feel better physically and emotionally, and become "new" polio survivors.

Twenty Million More

The story of polio and the facts about the cause, treatment, and management of PPS need to reach every polio survivor and every doctor, because twenty million polio survivors across the globe need their new symptoms to be believed and need help in treating them.

But there are thirty million more individuals throughout the world who have disabling conditions and can also benefit from polio survivors' painful experiences and our new knowledge about the late effects of polio. There are clear parallels dating from as far back as 1935 between polio and what in the 1980s came to be called chronic fatigue syndrome. These parallels can help us understand, treat, and manage CFS as well as fibromyalgia—both conditions affecting millions of people worldwide in which doctors also choose not to believe. Twenty million more individuals with a variety of disabilities—cerebral palsy, spina bifida, Guillain-Barre syndrome, and spinal cord injury—are also experiencing fatigue, muscle weakness, and pain in midlife, and seeing their abilities ebb away. They too have much to learn from polio survivors' experiences.

So come and meet some of the world's twenty million polio survivors, listen to their stories, and learn the important lessons they are eager to teach. Whether you had polio, have chronic fatigue syndrome, fibromyalgia, or are suffering the slings and arrows of aging with any disability, the lessons polio survivors have learned—about their bodies and their minds, about disability, society, and the way medicine is practiced—must be applied to everyone. Only then can we all survive and thrive in this new century as polio survivors learned to survive and thrive in the last.

CHAPTER 2

Once and Again

It was cold and windy on that northern New Jersey night in 1981 as I arrived for dinner at Susan's house. The few remaining leaves clattered across the sidewalk, driven by a raw wind that made my ankles ache. In fact I ached all over, especially the muscle on the top of my left leg. And I was tired, more tired than I could ever remember.

Susan's house had a lot of exterior concrete steps that had always pushed the outside of my stair-climbing envelope. I felt more exhausted than triumphant on reaching the front door; the struggle to climb each step raised a wrenching question I had never had to ask before: "Can I climb the inside stairs?" Susan greeted me happily as I faced Mount Suribachi. Before I reached the fourth step, I knew if I tried even one more my left leg would buckle and I would go down. As I explained my predicament to Susan, I started to cry. As she helped me to sit, I was terrified. I had no idea what was happening to me. Why couldn't I do tonight what I had been able to do for thirty years?

Unable to walk up the inside stairway, I bumped up the remaining steps on my behind, just as I had done in my parents' inaccessible home when I was a child. I pulled myself across the floor and, with Susan's help, was able to stand and shakily walked on my crutches to the dinner table.

After dinner I put on a brave face for Susan. I don't remember how I got down all of those stairs but I did, somehow, and was able to drive home, where I had an emotional meltdown. My entire world felt like it was spinning out of control. I felt completely vulnerable in a world where I had carved out my own productive and very independent niche. I had climbed thousands upon thousands of stairs in college and graduate school and had held a series of more and more responsible jobs. I had never let my body stop me. But I couldn't go to work the next day. I was afraid to leave my apartment for fear my legs would fail me again.

I did return to work, still afraid, still wondering what was happening to me. I knew no one else who had had polio. There was no one to ask, "You having trouble climbing stairs lately?" But even if I had known another polio survivor, I wouldn't have called. It never occurred to me that my leg weakness and increasing fatigue possibly could be connected to my polio thirty-two years before. I also didn't connect the yearlong muscle spasm in my leg to my inability to climb those stairs.

But I could no longer ignore the fact that something radically new and unwelcome was happening to my body. I suspect every polio survivor has their "Moment of Truth." Susan's stairway was mine.

NANCY, CLASS OF '49

And so it began. From New Jersey to New Mexico, from New Brunswick to New South Wales, thousands upon thousands of polio survivors were beginning to realize in the early 1980s that something radically new and unwelcome was happening to their bodies. But why, when there is evidence that the poliovirus has been around since at least the time of the pharaohs, did it take until 1980 for polio survivors to report that fatigue, weakness, and pain were occurring years after their bout with polio? Truth be told, the problems Nancy experienced in 1981 had been reported at least 106 years before.

The French Patient

In 1875 an unusual case was presented to the Society of Biology in Paris. A nineteen-year-old patient had had polio when he was six months old that paralyzed his left side. The young man had recovered partial use of his left arm and leg and became a tanner, which required him to use his arms to pull heavy, wet hides out of vats of acid. By the time he was seventeen, this French patient reported fatigue and a feeling of heaviness in his right arm, the arm that had apparently *not* been affected by the polio. His right arm and leg both became weaker and smaller. On hearing this presentation, the renowned French neurologist Jean Martin Charcot concluded that the young tanner's new weakness was due to overusing his stronger right arm, damage done by the poliovirus somehow having "moved" from the left side of his body to the right.

That same year, three other French doctors described other polio survivors who had developed muscle weakness and atrophy, a shrinking of the muscles, fifteen to almost thirty years after they had had polio. From 1875 until 1900, twenty-four articles appeared in European medical journals describing thirty additional polio survivors experiencing new weakness and sometimes atrophy—muscle shrinking—in limbs that obviously had been affected during the polio attack, but also in limbs that had apparently been unaffected. In 1899 British doctor William Hirsch reviewed all the cases reported during the nineteenth century. He concluded that there were three possible causes for late-onset weakness in polio survivors:

• The poliovirus had damaged spinal cord motor neurons—the cells that make muscles contract—making them vulnerable to some other disease later in life.
• Certain individuals were susceptible to developing motor neuron diseases, a susceptibility that allowed them to get polio as children and then develop another disease called "progressive muscular atrophy" later in life.
• Spinal cord motor neurons had been "scarred" by the

poliovirus, setting the stage for a "flare-up" at a later date, which caused new weakness.

Hirsch was the first to suggest that the poliovirus could somehow damage neurons early in life, damage that somehow caused new muscle weakness many years later.

In 1903 Charles Potts wrote the twentieth century's first article on the late effects of polio—the first to appear in an American medical journal—in which he too reviewed the nineteenth-century cases. Potts concluded that two of the polio survivors described had ALS—amyotrophic lateral sclerosis, which would come to be called Lou Gehrig's disease—a fatal disease that causes progressive paralysis of muscles throughout the body as a result of the death of the spinal cord motor neurons. However, Potts added that the overwhelming majority of the polio survivors described thus far in the medical journals did not have ALS but instead had progressive muscular atrophy Hirsch had mentioned, a disease of unknown origin that damages the spinal cord motor neurons, causes muscles to become weaker and smaller, but is not fatal.

From 1903 until the year of Nancy's frightening moment of truth, nearly two dozen additional articles were published that described late-onset symptoms in scores of polio survivors. In 1936 New York neurologists Salmon and Riley were the first to report that late-onset muscle weakness was not necessarily progressive and permanent but could be "transitory," with muscle strength decreasing and then increasing again after a period of time. Salmon and Riley agreed with Charles Potts that polio survivors were developing progressive muscular atrophy, suggesting that the poliovirus "may affect only slightly certain nerve cells or even lie dormant in the nervous system for an indefinite length of time and only at some later date make its presence known." Thus Salmon and Riley introduced two new ideas. The first was that slight damage, insufficient to cause muscle weakness during the polio attack, could somehow "make its presence known" later, explaining why polio survivors were reporting weakness in muscles that had apparently been unaffected by polio. The second was the new and frightening notion that the poliovirus might lie dormant in the spinal cord and somehow cause muscle weakness decades later.

The dearth of articles between 1936 and 1960 about late effects in polio survivors is undoubtedly due to polio's incidence reaching epidemic proportions. All of medicine was focused on dealing with the acute problems being experienced by the hundreds of thousands of individuals infected with the poliovirus during those years, and on developing a polio vaccine. But articles about late-onset problems appeared again. A 1962 British paper by K. J. Zilkha was the first to follow the course of muscle weakness in polio survivors over many years. He reported that although polio survivors did become weaker with time, they did not develop an inability to swallow and breathe, the life-threatening muscle paralysis characteristic of ALS. In 1964 Italian neurologists Pinelli and Ramelli reviewed all of the existing articles and proposed yet another possible cause for new muscle weakness. They noted that the motor neurons surviving the poliovirus attack send out new "sprouts"—like extra branches of a tree or new telephone wires—to activate muscle fibers orphaned when their motor neurons were killed. They suggested that new muscle weakness could result when overgrown motor neurons were unable to nourish and activate all of those extra "branches," and the sprouts died.

In 1970 three British lung specialists reported on fifty-five of their own polio patients who were experiencing not only muscle weakness but also "excessive fatigue," "breathlessness," an inability to concentrate, drowsiness, and "severe attacks of sleepiness." These patients also reported "abnormal sensitivity to cold especially of the extremities." Not surprisingly, the doctors found that treating polio survivors' breathing problems decreased their symptoms. However, it was noteworthy, that 90 percent of the patients with new symptoms had no problems with breathing. Also important was their conclusion that "highly motivated patients who pushed themselves beyond the competence" of their damaged bodies were most likely to develop late-onset problems.

And in 1980 a group of Italian doctors described their own post-polio patients and reviewed all the cases described since that French tanner reported fatigue and muscle weakness back in 1875. They concluded that although only one hundred cases had been described in the preceding 105 years, late-onset problems in polio survivors were "far from being rare." They agreed that polio survivors can develop new muscle weakness in obviously affected as well as "apparently spared" limbs, and that late-onset symptoms represented a "new process distinguishable from the old disease."

So when Nancy experienced her frightening moment of truth, she was far from alone. She just didn't know it. One hundred polio survivors had been described in the world's medical literature reporting the same symptoms. As Nancy lay terrified in her bed, her body failing her, untold thousands of polio survivors around the world were having the same experience. What *was* known on that cold and windy night in 1981? More than a hundred years of observation had taught that years after the polio attack:

• Polio survivors experience weakness, either transient or permanent, both in muscles obviously affected by polio and in those that had apparently been unaffected.

• Polio survivors experience excessive fatigue, an inability to concentrate, drowsiness, and sometimes severe attacks of sleepiness.

• Polio survivors' limbs are abnormally sensitive to cold.

• Polio survivors do become weaker over time, but are not developing the progressive and fatal disease ALS.

• Polio survivors like Nancy who are highly motivated, who push themselves "beyond the competence" of their polio-damaged bodies, are most likely to develop new symptoms.

What *wasn't* known on that night in 1981? It wasn't known *why* polio survivors were experiencing new symptoms. Were they developing a new motor neuron disease, a progressive muscular atrophy? Was slight damage to poliovirus-infected neurons somehow "flaring up" to cause weakness in muscles that had apparently been unaffected by polio? Were oversprouted motor neurons breaking apart because they were unable to nourish and activate their extra sprouts? Worst of all, could poliovirus lie dormant in the body and somehow become reactivated to cause new symptoms decades after the original poliovirus infection? We needed answers to all these questions if we were to understand what was happening to Nancy and to her fellow polio survivors and just what we had to do to treat their new symptoms.

To begin to answer these questions we need to return to the *locus in quo,* the scene of the crime, to understand what the poliovirus did inside the body and how it was able to enter, damage, and kill neurons. We also need to know how infected neurons were able not only to survive an onslaught by the poliovirus but also to recover and function again. Finally, we need to ask what it was about having polio that caused polio survivors to push themselves "beyond the competence of their damaged bodies," and how that pushing caused them to develop new symptoms.

First, then, to the scene of the crime.

The Guided Missile

The average number of spinal cord motor neurons that are destroyed by the poliovirus is almost 50 percent. However, non-paralytic polio may be associated with severe neuron damage in the spinal cord. What is more, some with non-paralytic poliomyelitis do not have any damage in the spinal cord but have characteristic damage in the brain, which is more extensive than in some who did have paralysis. All available evidence shows conclusively that every case of polio exhibits damage in the brain. The poliovirus is capable of producing an encephalitis, with or without symptoms, in the absence of any damage to the spinal cord. As far as the pathologist is concerned all cases of polio are "encephalitic."

PATHOLOGIST DAVID BODIAN

It has always amazed me that most polio survivors have no idea what the poliovirus is and what damage it did inside their bodies. To understand the cause, treatment, and management of PPS, we need to understand how and where the poliovirus did its dirty deeds: how it got into the body and into neurons and damaged them, and where in the spinal cord and brain that damage

occurred. What's more, we need to understand how damage
done during the poliovirus attack set the stage for the development of new symptoms decades later, and what that damage
means in terms of treating those symptoms.

The Missile Itself

It's amazing that something so small can do so much damage.
The poliovirus is only one-millionth of an inch across. About seventeen thousand poliovirus particles would cover the period at
the end of this sentence.

Each individual poliovirus particle looks like a soccer ball, its
surface made up of fifteen interconnecting "plates."

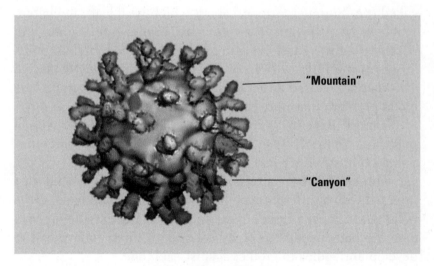

THE POLIOVIRUS

Each plate has "mountains" rising outward, and these create
"canyons" on the virus surface. The canyons are important
because they are where the poliovirus attaches itself to cells in
your body. But the poliovirus doesn't attach to and damage just
any cell. It is a "guided missile" that does one thing: seek out,

damage, and destroy the neurons that "activate" you—the ones that activate your brain and muscles. The poliovirus is the perfect human "OFF switch."

And there isn't just one poliovirus. There are three different types, each named for the location where it was found, either in a city or inside a person: Brunhilde, Lansing, and Leon. The three types are different because your immune system makes a different antibody for each. But they are also different in terms of how common they are and their ability to cause harm. Almost all of history's polio epidemics have been the result of Type I poliovirus, which caused leg, arm, and sometimes breathing muscle paralysis. The Type II virus seems to have been least likely to cause paralysis but may have damaged the "stem" at the bottom of the brain, just above the spinal cord, and was responsible for huge outbreaks of "nonparalytic" polio and something called the "Summer Grippe," about which we'll learn in chapter 17. Type III poliovirus, the most rare, also caused leg and arm paralysis but was most likely to produce so-called "bulbar" polio, in which the bulb or stem of the brain was severely damaged. This damage caused difficulties with swallowing, breathing, and blood pressure that were sometimes fatal.

It's most likely that you were infected with only one type of poliovirus, probably Type I, which caused all of your symptoms. Some polio survivors had two types at the same time, while a very unlucky few were attacked by one type in one year and then infected with a different type later in life. You could have gotten polio twice or even three times, because in the days before vaccine the body needed to be exposed to all three polioviruses to develop antibodies to protect against each one.

Even though there are only three types of poliovirus, there are at least fifty variations of the types, called strains. The existence of different strains has nothing to do with antibodies but everything to do with virulence, strains' differing ability to multiply in your body, to get inside your neurons and damage them. The fact that some poliovirus strains actually do little or no damage to your neurons allowed Albert Sabin to develop a polio vaccine that contains all three types of polioviruses that are live but non-virulent, that is, able to cause your body to produce antibodies, but unable to get inside your neurons to do damage. The existence of dozens of different poliovirus strains makes it clear that polioviruses mutate inside people and can change their virulence. In fact, experiments in animals show that the passage of poliovirus—infecting one animal with a poliovirus, having that animal infect another, and so on—can increase virulence. As the polioviruses passed from person to person during the middle of the twentieth century, they apparently became more virulent, causing more paralysis and killing more people in 1950 than they did in 1920, a story that I'll tell in the next chapter.

Over the Teeth and Past the Gums

The first question you may ask is how you came to be infected with any of the polioviruses. No, it wasn't spoiled milk, filthy flies, or being mean to your sister. The polioviruses belong to a nasty family of seventy-two viruses called enteroviruses, so named because they grow in your "entrails," your intestines. You were infected with the poliovirus when you came in close contact with someone who was already infected and some of his or her saliva or intestinal secretions found their way into your mouth. From there the poliovirus went on a ten-day, unnoticed tour of your insides. It first moved into the spongy tissue of your tonsils and began to multiply. While poliovirus was growing in back of your throat, it also moved downward, into and through your stomach, and reached your small intestine. There it entered Peyer's patches, miniature cavelike lymph nodes in the wall of the intestine, which provided a warm and welcoming way station in which the poliovirus multiplied like mad. Also inside the Peyer's patches are white blood cells called monocytes—the same cells of which you have too many if you get mononucleosis. Sticking up from the surface of the monocytes are structures essential for the poliovirus to do its dirty deeds: poliovirus receptors, miniature proteins that look like crooked fingers and fit perfectly into those canyons on the surface of the virus.

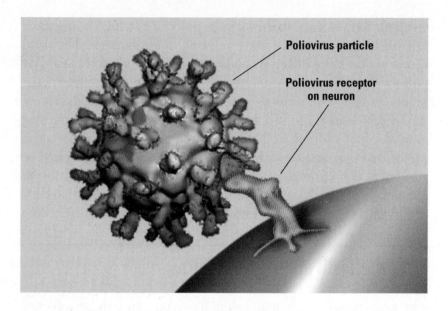

Poliovirus particle

Poliovirus receptor on neuron

POLIOVIRUS AND RECEPTOR

Receptors on monocytes hooked the poliovirus and pulled it inside, where it also multiplied. Meanwhile, when so much poliovirus was produced in your tonsils that it could no longer be contained there, it flowed back into the throat, mixed with saliva, and made you capable of infecting someone else. Large amounts of poliovirus and infected monocytes were released from Peyer's patches back into the intestines, too, and passed out with the intestinal contents, also making it possible for you to pass polio to someone else.

Poliovirus released from both the tonsils and intestines also traveled to the large lymph nodes under your arms, where it multiplied even further. Finally, about ten days after you were infected, when your largest lymph nodes could no longer contain the millions upon millions of poliovirus particles, huge amounts of virus spilled into your bloodstream. Your blood, full of poliovirus and virus-infected monocytes, carried its deadly cargo toward its intended destination: the neurons in your brain and spinal cord.

Entrez Vous, Brunhilde

Virus-laden blood flowed up into your head and found "leaky" places in the brain's blood vessels; where poliovirus flowed into the brain. At the same time, infected monocytes passed through the walls of brain blood vessels, acting like "poliovirus taxis" that also allowed virus to enter the brain. Once inside, poliovirus latched on to poliovirus receptors, found on the surface of neurons in the brain stem and on motor neurons, within both the brain and the spinal cord.

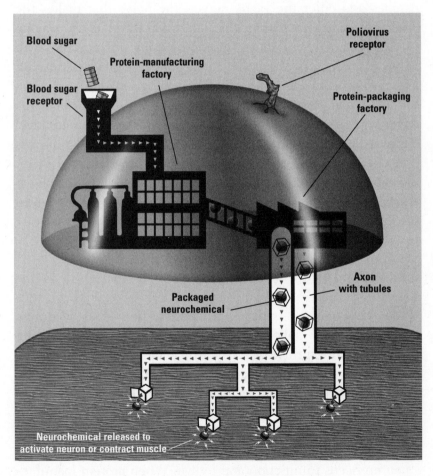

NEURON BEFORE POLIOVIRUS ATTACK

Once inside those neurons, the poliovirus multiplied, infected other nearby brain neurons, and also traveled inside neurons to penetrate more deeply into the brain. Then the poliovirus could head south, descending inside spinal cord neurons and ending up in the motor neurons that control the muscles of your diaphragm, neck, back, arms, and legs, where it also multiplied and infected other nearby spinal cord neurons.

There's yet a third way poliovirus could reach brain and spinal cord motor neurons: backward. Viruses that multiply in the intestines, such as the poliovirus, can flow out of the Peyer's patches and enter the vagus nerve—the nerve that makes the intestines contract—inside which they can travel all the way up to the brain. What's more, motor neurons are covered with poliovirus receptors where they make contact with your muscles. When your blood was full of virus, damaging a muscle and puncturing a blood vessel could bathe neurons with virus. Poliovirus receptors could pull virus into the neurons, where it could travel backward into the spinal cord and brain. In chapter 4 I'll discuss that children whose muscles had been slightly damaged by an injection were up to ten times more likely to get paralytic polio—and were most often paralyzed in the limb where they received the injection.

The Dirty Deeds

Once the poliovirus reaches a neuron, how does it do its damage? After a poliovirus receptor latches on, it pulls the poliovirus to the surface of the neuron and causes it to "unzip"—releasing its contents inside the neuron. And this is when the cycle of destruction begins. Inside each poliovirus particle are about a dozen individual proteins that do the dirty deeds. These proteins are enzymes that shut down and then literally break apart the "factories" that manufacture and package the proteins a neuron needs to function and to live. When protein manufacturing is stopped, the neuron can no longer make neurochemi-

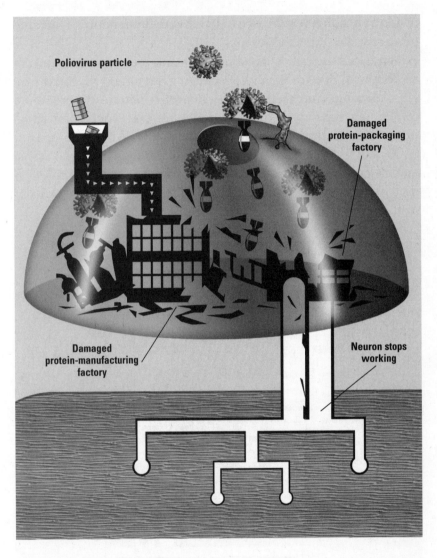

Poliovirus particle

Damaged
protein-packaging
factory

Damaged
protein-manufacturing
factory

Neuron stops
working

POLIOVIRUS-INFECTED NEURON

cals—the proteins that allow one neuron to talk to another and
that allow motor neurons to make muscles contract. When neurochemicals stop being made, the neuron's OFF switch is thrown.

Muscles become weaker or are paralyzed; brain neurons become less active or stop functioning.

Why does the poliovirus shut down and break apart a neuron's protein-manufacturing and -packaging factories? Because the virus uses bits and pieces of the neuron's factories to create its own poliovirus production plant, which constructs thousands upon thousands of new poliovirus particles. When the neuron totally fills with virus, it explodes and dies, releasing massive quantities of poliovirus that travel to other neurons, bind with their poliovirus receptors, causing the whole destructive process to start again.

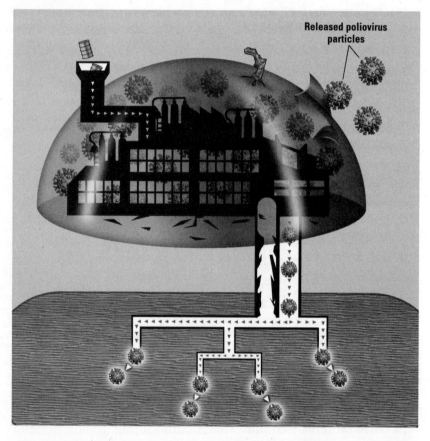

NEURONS BECOME POLIOVIRUS–MANUFACTURING FACTORIES

The Numbers Game

The poliovirus is remarkable in its ability to invade neurons. In the 1940s Johns Hopkins University pathologist David Bodian found that 96 percent of motor neurons were infected by the poliovirus if you had any paralysis at all! Given the ability of poliovirus to enter and damage such a large percentage of neurons, why doesn't everyone infected with poliovirus become totally and permanently paralyzed? Bodian found that for each neuron the poliovirus invades, commandeers, and destroys, its action is halted in another neuron that is then able to rebuild its severely damaged protein-manufacturing and protein-packaging factories and start functioning again. How is it that the poliovirus is stopped at least half the time? Most likely because the immune system is able to play catch-up and produce enough antibodies to attack the poliovirus before it conquers the entire nervous system.

But if on average 50 percent of all motor neurons are destroyed in anyone who had paralytic polio, why aren't half of polio survivors' muscles paralyzed? Bodian discovered that at least 60 percent of spinal cord motor neurons associated with an individual muscle must be killed before the muscle shows any weakness at all. This means that muscles that were at one time paralyzed, or muscles that have always been weak, may be operating on as few as 40 percent of their original motor neurons. It's as if you had a ten-cylinder car before you had polio and have a four-cylinder car afterward—a car that has driven just fine for forty years or more. What's more, Bodian found that muscles thought to be completely unaffected by polio—muscles that had never been weak, let alone paralyzed—only have 60 percent of their original motor neurons. Think about it. The muscles you thought the poliovirus had spared are running on only six of the ten motor neurons they originally had. Your seemingly unaffected muscles are running on only six cylinders.

Knowing these percentages is pivotal to an understanding of

the cause, treatment, and management of PPS, and leads to the first Post-Polio Precept:

THERE IS NO SUCH THING AS AN UNAFFECTED MUSCLE IF ANY MUSCLE WAS AFFECTED BY POLIO.

This precept is a reminder that you need to take care of the muscles you thought escaped the original poliovirus onslaught as well as those you know were affected.

Plugged Plumbing

Unfortunately, there's even more to the aftermath of polio than losing about half of your motor neurons. What happened to the neurons that were invaded and damaged but did not die? The surviving motor neurons rebuilt their protein factories and started functioning again. Remarkably, this internal rebuilding process took only about a month. So you might have been paralyzed during the polio attack—when the virus took over, killed off, and shut down motor neurons—but still walked out of the hospital a month or so later, after the surviving, infected neurons rebuilt their protein factories and started functioning again.

However, those recovered neurons were never the same as they were before the poliovirus invaded. Damaged and rebuilt neurons are smaller and also have shrunken axons—the cable-like extensions that travel out sometimes for several feet from spinal cord motor neurons to connect with muscles.

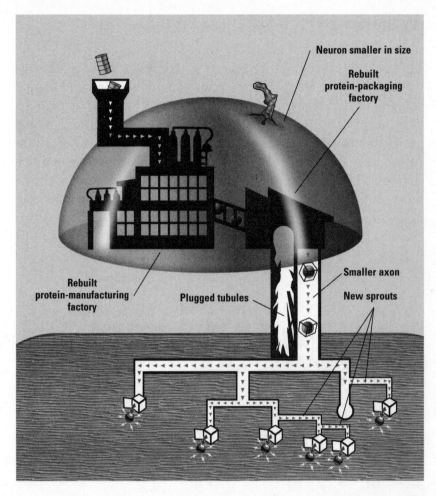

SURVIVING AND FUNCTIONING POST-POLIO NEURON

What's more, the microscopic tubules within the neurons were "plugged" with debris that was probably created when the poliovirus broke apart the neurons' innards. Like clogged pipes, plugged tubules can't carry all the proteins, nutrients, and neurochemicals where they need to go inside the neuron. So not only do polio survivors have fewer motor neurons, but also the remaining neurons are damaged in ways that decrease their ability to talk to other neurons and make muscles move.

Axons Sprouts and Fat Fibers

This post-infection picture sounds pretty bleak. But there's also good news. The remaining, damaged motor neurons did something amazing after the poliovirus infection had run its course. The axons grew, sending out sprouts—like extra telephone lines—to turn on the muscles that were orphaned when their motor neurons were killed. Those sprouts took from nine months to two years to grow, and ultimately activated about sixteen times more muscle fibers than were connected to the motor neuron originally.

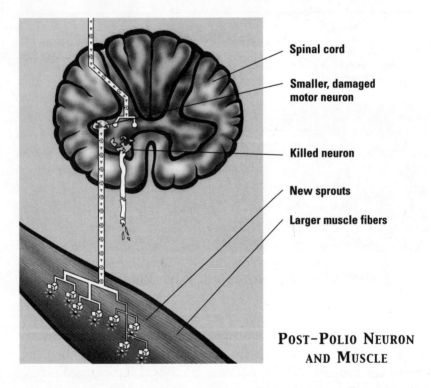

Spinal cord

Smaller, damaged motor neuron

Killed neuron

New sprouts

Larger muscle fibers

**POST-POLIO NEURON
AND MUSCLE**

Yet another important process took place that allowed polio survivors to regain strength. Muscle-strengthening exercise and physical therapy caused muscle fibers to grow larger, a process called hypertrophy, enabling the fibers to do more work. Polio survivors' individual muscle fibers have been found to be about twice the size of fibers in those who've never had polio. Thus motor neuron recovery, sprouting, and muscle fiber hypertrophy allowed polio survivors to get stronger after the poliovirus attack. A 1955 study by British polio pioneer W. J. W. Sharrard found that polio survivors regained nearly 95 percent of the strength they would ever recover during the first eleven months after the polio attack as a result of sprouting, muscle fiber hypertrophy, and learning to use functioning muscles to substitute for those that were permanently paralyzed.

So where do you stand (or sit) today with regard to your post-polio motor neurons? If you had any paralysis, muscles that you know were affected during the poliovirus attack now have on average only 40 percent of the motor neurons you were born with. What's more, the neurons you do have were damaged, are smaller than normal, and have clogged internal pipes, but have also sprouted to turn on sixteen times more muscle fibers— fibers on average twice the size they were before you had polio. If you have muscles that were not paralyzed or had so-called "nonparalytic" polio, you have on average only 60 percent of the motor neurons you were born with, neurons that were damaged and are smaller, clogged, oversprouted, and overworked.

The Main Event

The damage to spinal cord motor neurons we've been discussing is called "poliomyelitis." In Latin *polio* means "gray," while *myelitis* refers to an inflammation of the neurons in the spinal cord. Gray neurons are those not covered in myelin, the white, fatty insulation that separates one neuron from another. *Poliomyelitis* is the fancy name generally applied to any infection by the poliovirus. You may have heard a doctor or your parents say that you had poliomyelitis. And if you had paralysis or muscle weakness, you certainly did have myelitis, an inflammation of the motor neurons in the spinal cord. Still, the name *poliomyelitis* shouldn't be applied to everyone infected by the poliovirus, because inflammation of the spinal cord did not always occur. Poliomyelitis was actually an afterthought of the poliovirus. In fact, the main event of the poliovirus attack was not in the spinal cord at all.

BODIAN'S PARADOX

This chapter began with the comments of a remarkable scientist, pathologist David Bodian. Bodian is the unsung hero of polio and PPS. It was he who discovered that there are three types of poliovirus. By performing scores of autopsies on animals and people who had polio, Bodian also uncovered the path the poliovirus followed—from the intestines, to the lymph nodes, and into the blood—that ultimately ended with infection of your neurons. Bodian's discovery that the poliovirus entered the blood before it entered the neurons made a polio vaccine possible.

Autopsies also allowed David Bodian to determine that the poliovirus damaged neurons' protein factories, as well as just how many neurons on average were damaged and killed during an attack. This work revealed that the main event of poliovirus infection was not myelitis—not an inflammation of spinal cord motor neurons—but an *encephalitis*, an inflammation of the brain. In every case of polio Bodian studied, paralytic and "non-paralytic," he saw a consistent pattern of damage to brain neurons. Bodian's findings reveal another Polio Paradox, this time in the form of a statement "contrary to received opinion":

IN ALL CASES OF POLIO "AN ENCEPHALITIS EXISTS WHETHER SYMPTOMS ARE PRESENT OR NOT."

If we are to understand all the damage done by the poliovirus and explain the cause of PPS symptoms other than muscle weakness, we must understand the important implications of Bodian's Paradox: that the poliovirus is in fact a guided missile aimed directly at the brain.

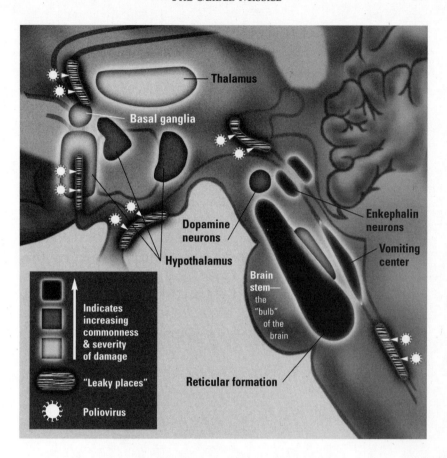

Thalamus

Basal ganglia

Dopamine
neurons

Hypothalamus

Enkephalin
neurons

Vomiting
center

Brain
stem—
the
"bulb"
of the
brain

Indicates
increasing
commonness
& severity
of damage

"Leaky places"

Poliovirus

Reticular formation

POLIOVIRUS DAMAGE TO THE BRAIN

BURNING OUT THE BULB

The most common and severe poliovirus damage revealed by
Bodian's autopsies was at the bottom of the brain, in the brain
stem or "bulb" of the brain. Bodian found that the brain stem
was "involved in even mild cases" of polio. The brain stem contains the reticular formation, a netlike web of neurons that is
responsible for automatically activating both your brain and your
body. The reticular formation sends signals upward to activate

the cortex, the "supercomputer" of the brain, to keep you awake and to focus your attention. The reticular formation also sends signals downward through the spinal cord to automatically tell your diaphragm to move up and down, to control your blood pressure and heart rate, the muscles in your throat, and to maintain muscle tone. Polio patients who had severe damage to the brain stem could not swallow or breathe on their own because the reticular formation neurons could not tell the muscles to contract. Some survivors were placed in iron lungs that moved the diaphragm and would breathe for them. These individuals were diagnosed as having "bulbar" polio, because the poliovirus did such obvious damage to neurons in the "bulb" of the brain. It was this severe damage to reticular formation neurons that made polio a killer. But it's important to remember that *every* polio survivor, with or without obvious swallowing or breathing problems, had "bulbar" polio, since the reticular formation was the one area of the brain Bodian found was always damaged by the poliovirus.

ONWARD AND UPWARD

Once the poliovirus entered the brain, it could travel downward and enter the spinal cord motor neurons to cause poliomyelitis with its arm and leg paralysis. In addition, the poliovirus traveled upward to attack brain neurons that also participate in the process of making muscles move. The poliovirus damaged and killed neurons in the basal ganglia, which both start and stop muscle movement, and neurons that make dopamine, the neurochemical that activates the basal ganglia. The poliovirus actually traveled all the way up to the neurons in your cortex, where the signal that tells a muscle to move originates. Remarkably, the poliovirus damaged only cortical motor neurons. For example, when David Bodian actually injected poliovirus directly into monkeys' vision neurons at the back of their brains, absolutely nothing happened; the neurons kept working! The polioviruses' lack of interest in any neurons other than cortical motor neurons prevented polio survivors from having any impairment in their ability to think. However another important brain function was affected by the polioviruses' northern road trip.

As poliovirus traveled upward, brain-activating neurons in addition to those in the reticular formation were attacked. Neurons in the basal ganglia and those that make dopamine not only are involved in muscle movement, but also play an important role in activating the entire brain. Dopamine is in fact the principal brain-activating neurochemical (I'll have much more to say about dopamine in chapter 11). Other brain-activating neurons were killed by the poliovirus, including those in the hypothalamus, the brain center that automatically controls the body's internal environment, and the thalamus, the central relay station that directs information to the cortex. With so much damage to brain-activating neurons, it's no surprise that polioencephalitis was associated with drowsiness, prolonged sleeping, attention deficits—sometimes even coma—whether or not there was poliomyelitis or any muscle paralysis.

The Aftermath and the Prelude

So that's the story of the guided missile. But the poliovirus and the damage it did to the brain and spinal cord is only the beginning of the tale. We need to go farther if we're to understand all that happened to those attacked by the poliovirus. What caused polio to become epidemic in the middle of the last century? Why did some people get polio while others were spared? How many people were attacked by the poliovirus? To answer these questions, let's return to those frightening days of yesteryear.

CHAPTER 4

An Awesome Thing

New York Journal, June 27, 1916. The strange epidemic which has caused fourteen deaths during the month is attributed by doctors to the prolonged damp weather of this spring and early summer. More than one hundred persons from Brooklyn are suffering from it, and it is said to be epidemic from Bridgeport to Philadelphia.

"This was the first marked public consciousness of an epidemic of infantile paralysis that was to sweep over the northeastern section of the United States before the fateful summer of 1916 had passed, leaving 27,000 persons— mostly children—victims of the dread disease and killing more than 6,000 of them. New York City with its teeming millions in congested slum areas took a heavy blow, the score finally standing at more than 9,000 victims, almost all children; 2,000 dead, and the majority of those surviving crippled for life."

RONALD BERG, 1948

The poliovirus is an awesome thing. It has sickened, disabled, and killed countless millions of people since it first appeared in . . . well, truth be told, we have no idea where polio first

appeared. The first known image of a polio survivor was carved
in stone in the tomb of an Egyptian priest named Rom circa
1580 B.C. Rom is shown with a "withered limb and dropped foot"
that any polio survivor today would recognize in a compatriot.
About a thousand years later, another polio survivor was portrayed in the painting *The Procession of Cripples*.

The lack of more frequent depictions of polio survivors is evidence of an important fact: Throughout human history, paralytic
polio has been the exception, not the rule. The only reason we're
talking about PPS today is because the poliovirus attacked millions of people during the middle of the twentieth century. The
first question we have to answer to explain the emergence of
PPS is why there have been polio epidemics at all.

Wherefore Polio Epidemics?

If you read any textbook on infectious diseases, you'll come
across what epidemiologist Neal Nathanson calls the "Central
Dogma" of polio. The Central Dogma states that the poliovirus,
to have survived throughout the ages, must have lived inside lots
of people because its only natural habitat is the human intestine.
And given that large amounts of poliovirus pass out of the body
with the contents of the intestine, it is thought that open sewers
and infrequent hand washing in the eons before indoor
plumbing allowed poliovirus to readily pass from person to
person. But if virtually everyone was infected by the poliovirus,
the fact that polio epidemics were the exception and not the rule
until the twentieth century yields another Polio Paradox:

**POLIO EPIDEMICS DID NOT OCCUR PRECISELY BECAUSE
EVERYONE WAS INFECTED WITH THE POLIOVIRUS.**

How could this possibly be true? Newborn babies survive in a
world teeming with viruses and bacteria because mothers pass to
their children antibodies against bugs to which moms have been
exposed. Mothers' antibodies, which enter babies' blood when

they are in the womb, protect infants until they're about six months old. Throughout history, it was during those six months—while being protected against the damaging effects of the poliovirus by Mom's antibodies—that infants were infected with the virus because of poor sanitation and poor personal hygiene. According to the Central Dogma, then, for thousands of years infants were "vaccinated" against polio during early infancy by the poliovirus itself, and received "booster" vaccinations throughout their lives through additional exposure. Only rare individuals would not have received their mother's antibodies or would not have been exposed to poliovirus during those first six protected months. They would not have developed their own immunity, would have been susceptible to the poliovirus, and would have been paralyzed, as was Rom.

Why then did polio epidemics ever appear? Good grooming at the dawn of the twentieth century, according to the Central Dogma, which states that the cause of polio epidemics was "improvements in public sanitation and personal hygiene" occurring around 1880. With the advent of indoor plumbing, people no longer had intimate and prolonged contact with poliovirus carried in the contents of their intestines. This meant that infants were no longer exposed to the poliovirus during those early months when they were protected by their mothers' antibodies and were not able to develop their own poliovirus antibodies. According to the Central Dogma, infants who came in contact with the poliovirus after their six months of maternal antibody protection ended were susceptible to a poliovirus attack. This is why three-quarters of those who contracted polio during the 1916 outbreak that decimated the Northeast were more than six months but less than five years old. This is why, in the early decades of the twentieth century, the disabling and often deadly disease caused by the poliovirus was called "Infantile Paralysis."

Is Cleanliness Next to Paralysis?

The Central Dogma has a problem: its basic premise, that central plumbing and hand washing reduced infants' exposure to poliovirus, thereby preventing development of antibodies and lifelong immunity during the first year of life. If poor hygiene in infancy had prevented polio epidemics for eons, then poor people with poor sanitation should have been protected against polio during the first epidemics around 1900. But this wasn't always true. As the *New York Journal* article said about the 1916 epidemic, "congested slum areas took a heavy blow." Indeed, New York City health commissioner Haven Emerson showed that immigrant New Yorkers, who were more likely to have been poor and living in congested slums, had nearly four times more polio than native-born Americans. The New York epidemic itself appears to have started in the Italian immigrant community. Across the Hudson River in Newark, New Jersey, the rate of polio was nearly *twice* that of New York City. Southern and eastern European immigrants, described as "junk dealers," "rag peddlers," and laborers, who lived in "unsanitary tenements" in the most congested parts of the city bore the brunt of Newark's epidemic.

So here's another Polio Paradox:

POLIO WAS SAID TO BE A DISEASE OF THE CLEANER MIDDLE CLASS, EVEN THOUGH THE FIRST BIG EPIDEMIC OCCURRED AMONG THE POOREST IMMIGRANTS.

We can look to epidemics that took place before and after 1916 to see if the Central Dogma or this Polio Paradox is correct—to see if good hygiene actually caused you to get polio.

Polio in America

The first American polio outbreak probably occurred in Louisiana in 1841. But the first sizable epidemics occurred in

New England in the early 1890s, the most notable striking Rutland County, Vermont, in 1884. One hundred children were paralyzed and many more were sickened.

In 1908 a small polio outbreak occurred in western Massachusetts. Public health doctor Herbert Emerson went house to house to see if he could identify factors responsible for the sixty-nine polio cases. He reported that "sanitary conditions" were "good to excellent" in only 30 percent of the households and "fair to bad" in 70 percent. "Water closets" were connected with the sewer in one-third of homes, while two-thirds had "earth closets." So in Massachusetts, most of those attacked by polio had poor sanitation.

Move ahead to 1935. The U.S. Public Health Service canvassed 200,000 American families in twenty-eight large cities. This door-to-door survey asked specifically whether any family member had ever had polio. It was estimated that there were 166,000 American polio survivors who had lasting paralysis, many of whom were part of the 1916 epidemic. Through this survey, statistician S. D. Collins painted the first detailed portrait of polio in America. He found that cases of polio peaked four weeks earlier in the South, around August 15, than in the North and West, where the peak was around September 15. Collins discovered that the typical age for polio was three years old; nearly three-quarters of those paralyzed were affected below the waist, just over half had only one foot or leg weakened, and in less than 10 percent were the arms involved. When polio affected only one leg, it affected the left twice as often as the right, even though 99 percent of polio survivors were right-handed.

With regard to poverty and cleanliness, Collins discovered that children under five years old on Relief (today's welfare) had almost 200 percent more polio than children in wealthier families. From 1938 to 1942 in Baltimore, Maryland, there was 40 percent more polio in children under five in the "lower class." In contradiction to the Central Dogma, poverty in infants and children, who were more likely to have poor hygiene, did not protect against polio. Collins did relate poverty to polio, but only in that poor people had "more contact in the crowded areas" of Baltimore, possibly the same reason New York's and Newark's poor immigrants in congested slum areas "took a heavy blow" in 1916. Even the last of the polio outbreaks, occurring after the Salk injectable polio vaccine became available in 1954, were largely urban and localized to "lower socioeconomic groups" living in crowded conditions. It makes sense that the closer together people live—especially if many share a common toilet—the more likely it is that poliovirus will pass easily from one person to another.

Polio Overseas

The Central Dogma of poverty and poor hygiene protecting against polio does not seem to hold true in other countries, either. In Europe polio flourished under conditions of terrible hygiene. The Netherlands' worst epidemic to date occurred in 1943 during the German occupation. After 1943 the frequency of polio decreased in the city of Amsterdam, a decrease thought to be remarkable by polio researcher Albert Sabin, who noted the "general severe underfeeding and the great deficiency of hygienic facilities." Sabin was also surprised that a large postwar epidemic occurred in Germany; to describe "bomb-blasted, congested Berlin [in 1947 as] unhygienic and extremely overcrowded is to put it mildly," he said. Yet polio flourished.

In reviewing these outbreaks, Sabin rejected the Central Dogma and the notion that improvements in public sanitation and personal hygiene prevented early exposure to poliovirus, prevented early immunization, and were therefore responsible for the polio epidemics. He suggested that "factors peculiar to certain regions, populations and groups [such as] way of life, soil, water, diet or environment"—and not merely lack of antibodies to poliovirus—were the causes of the epidemics, somehow making people susceptible to polio.

Region, Way of Life, and Environment

One peculiar factor Sabin related to the cause of polio epidemics
was region. Starting with the 1916 epidemic, polio in the United
States was a phenomenon of one region: the North. After 1916,
from coast to coast, the northern portion of the country experienced yearly late-summer outbreaks, with 1931 and 1935 being
banner years in the Northeast. However, in the South, there was
little polio until 1935. Then in 1941 the southeastern states
began to make up for lost time as cases of polio increased there
and throughout the country.

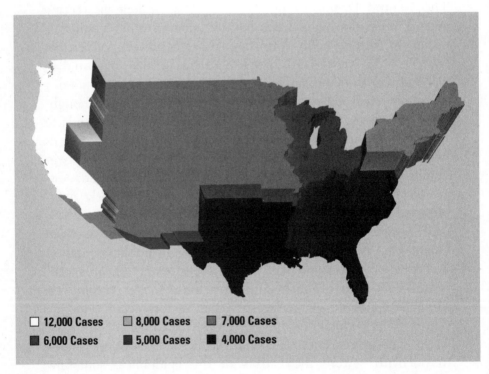

□ 12,000 Cases □ 8,000 Cases ■ 7,000 Cases
■ 6,000 Cases ■ 5,000 Cases ■ 4,000 Cases

REPORTED POLIO CASES BY REGION (1930–1944)

Why was there less polio in the South? Of course, the obvious explanation would be the Central Dogma: Southern poverty allowed poor hygiene, increased infants' exposure to poliovirus, and permitted them to develop antibodies early in life. But if the Central Dogma is rejected, what other factor might have prevented the South from experiencing the early polio epidemics that devastated the North? One possibility is the opposite of Collins's explanation for epidemics in the North: In the rural and much less densely populated South, people lived far apart and had less opportunity to pass the poliovirus from person to person.

Unfortunately, decreased exposure to poliovirus is a double-edged sword. Although people who are not exposed to poliovirus can't get polio, they also will never have an opportunity to develop antibodies. For example, after the 1955 polio epidemic in Iceland, poliovirus antibodies were found in 70 percent of children in the affected capital city, while none of the children in rural areas had antibodies. In the United States rural southerners may also have had less opportunity to be exposed to poliovirus and develop antibodies.

A lack of antibodies in southerners may explain the increase in polio not only in the South but also throughout the country during the 1930s and 1940s, when combined with significant changes in way of life, soil, water, and the environment. During those years the depression and the Dust Bowl forced farmers from Oklahoma and Arkansas to move west. It may not be a coincidence that one of the largest polio epidemics ever recorded occurred along the Pacific Coast in 1934 as southern farmers who may not have developed poliovirus antibodies poured into California, Washington, and Oregon.

It may also be no coincidence that polio epidemics began their unprecedented increase in 1942, the year America mobilized for World War II. The war brought even more migration, with southerners moving to northern cities to take war-related manufacturing jobs, and going off to war. The sudden appearance in the 1940s of epidemic polio in Africa along the overland route traveled by Allied troops from the Mideast to South Africa, was said to be due to the great movement and mixing of soldiers and civilians, causing increased opportunity for poor and very rural Africans to come in contact with poliovirus for the first time. After the war, more movement and mixing occurred as fifteen million men in uniform returned to the United States. No longer satisfied staying down on the farm, southerners moved to America's burgeoning cities. As early as the 1920s and continuing through the 1950s, the number of polio cases increased as more and more Americans moved into ever-more-crowded urban areas.

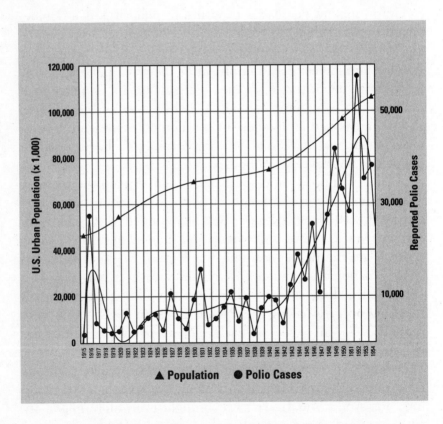

INCREASE IN REPORTED U.S. POLIO CASES WITH INCREASING URBAN POPULATION

So population density—and not poverty or cleanliness—may have been the spark that set off America's twentieth-century polio epidemics.

Groups and Populations

So far we've looked at three peculiar factors that Sabin thought might be fueling polio epidemics. One of those factors, the North–South regional divide, was also associated with a "group" factor: America's color divide. In Collins's survey almost 400 percent more white than African American children had polio in the Northeast; in the South about 25 percent more whites had polio than did African Americans. The striking difference in the number of white and African American polio survivors was used to support the Central Dogma. It was assumed that African Americans were poorer than whites, had poor hygiene, were exposed to poliovirus as infants, and developed immunity. The smaller difference in the percentage of white as compared to African American southern children who got polio also supported the Central Dogma, since all southerners were assumed to be poorer than northerners. Sabin rejected southern poverty as support for the Central Dogma, but he never specifically addressed the remarkably lower percentage of African Americans who got polio.

It is interesting to note that African American children in the Northeast had nearly 30 percent more polio than did black children in the South. Again, living in congested northeastern cities probably increased the likelihood of getting polio. Living in the rural and less populous South may have protected both blacks and whites against polio. Still, the fact remains that African Americans had less polio *everywhere* in America. It has always been remarkable to me that I have only met a handful of African American polio survivors during the past twenty years as I travel to speak at post-polio conferences in the North and the South. Also remarkable is that less than 3 percent of the patients we have treated over the past twenty years are African American, even though the percentage of African Americans in the U.S. population is about 11 percent. This poses a fascinating question. Could there be something about race, something in your genes, that makes you less—or more—likely to get polio?

RACIAL DIVIDES

Fascinating findings suggest that genetic factors do indeed predispose people to contracting polio. With regard to the color divide, the 1947 Casablanca epidemic saw nearly twenty times more polio among Europeans than native Africans. At the other end of the continent, during South Africa's 1948 epidemic four times more Europeans than native Africans had polio in large cities.

There are divides among other racial and ethnic groups. During the 1916 New York epidemic, Germanic and southern European immigrants had over 20 percent more polio than did immigrants from northern Europe and Great Britain, and had nearly 60 percent more polio than did those from eastern Europe. In Newark southern and eastern European immigrants were the hardest hit. No Asian immigrants were reported to have had polio.

The low rates of polio among Asians living in the East is also remarkable. During the early part of the twentieth century, paralytic polio was rare in China, Korea, and the Philippines. Albert Sabin was told by a British physician in northern China that he not infrequently saw paralytic polio in the children of foreigners but rarely saw the disease among natives. In 1946, although there was an outbreak of polio among American Marines stationed in northern China, not one case was reported among the Chinese. Polio also occurred with unexpected frequency in American servicemen stationed in the Philippines and Korea despite the fact that there had been no prior polio epidemics— and that even individual cases of polio among the local population were rare. In Hawaii, where there was no segregation of racial groups at all in terms of work, play, or housing, between 1938 and 1947 whites had almost three times more polio than did Japanese residents, at least four times more polio than Chinese residents, and nearly six times more polio than Hawaii's Filipino residents.

These findings suggest that one peculiar factor that predisposes to polio may be a gene associated with your racial or ethnic background. Apparently, the poliovirus has a peculiar affection for Germanic folk and southern Europeans. But might there be other genetic factors that have marked you for a poliovirus attack?

All in the Family

An obvious place to look for genetic factors that may predispose to polio is within families. In 5 to 20 percent of households where poliovirus attacked one family member, another was also stricken. From 1909 to 1955 more than two thousand family members were surveyed in over one thousand households in which at least one person had polio. Polio was thirteen times less common in those over twenty-five years old, so children were primarily affected. On average, if one child in a household became ill, he "shared" polio with one other sibling of similar age. (I say "he" because more boys contracted polio than did girls.) Just over half of those who became ill were paralyzed, while the others had flu-like symptoms ranging from a fever, sore throat, and nausea to a stiff neck and muscle pain. Such a "minor illness" was caused by the poliovirus but may never have been diagnosed as polio at all, or may have been called "abortive" or "nonparalytic" polio. In three-quarters of households the first case of polio was paralytic and the second "nonparalytic." The bottom line: There's about a one-in-five chance that if you had paralytic polio, one of your brothers or sisters had "nonparalytic" polio—and may not even have known it.

Unfortunately, these household studies could not separate the effect of sharing genes from sharing the same living space, the idea of "more contact in crowded areas" leading to greater exposure to the poliovirus and a greater likelihood of getting polio. But other studies have helped identify a genetic susceptibility to polio by tracing cases back through generations of family members who didn't necessarily share the same living quarters. H. V. Wyatt traced all of the cases of polio on the island of Malta from 1920 to 1964. Of more than a thousand cases during those decades, 80 percent of those who had polio were blood relatives. Studies from 1890 to the 1940s traced cases of polio back through several generations of Americans. Of nearly eight hundred polio survivors, almost 60 percent of polio cases occurred in relatives. The difference between Malta's 80 percent rate and the 60 percent rate seen in the United States may be the greater probability for close relatives to marry and have children on a small island, increasing the power of a "polio gene"; or it could be the result of more contact in a crowded area. But these studies still don't tell us just how much of your susceptibility to polio is genetic and how much comes from close contact to others who carry the virus.

TARHEEL TWINS

Three studies do help tease out the effect of genetic predisposition from poliovirus exposure. North Carolina doctor C. N. Herndon studied forty-five families in which polio affected twins. Herndon found that in 36 percent of identical twins (two people who shared the exact same genes), both were paralyzed by polio, while only 6 percent of fraternal twins (two people with genes no more similar than those of any two siblings) were both paralyzed. The percentage of polio in fraternal twins was similar to the 5 percent rate of polio in siblings of the twins. But since the twins and their brothers and sisters shared the same home, Herndon's findings still don't allow us to separate genetics from exposure.

As luck would have it, pioneering polio researcher Joseph

Melnick measured poliovirus antibodies before and after the big
1948 North Carolina epidemic, the worst in the state's history,
during which most of Herndon's twins had become ill. Melnick
found that 23 percent of North Carolinians were infected with
poliovirus but that only about 5 percent had any symptoms and
only 1 percent were paralyzed. Melnick's findings did away with
one Polio Fiction:

**EVERYONE INFECTED BY THE POLIOVIRUS
WILL BE PARALYZED.**

Combining Melnick's findings with Herndon's, since 1 percent of the general population and 6 percent of fraternal twins
and siblings living in the same household were paralyzed by
polio, living in close quarters increases the chance of getting
polio about sixfold. This increase is similar to that found in
studies of polio outbreaks in institutions, where people who were
not related lived in close quarters. The rate of polio in five resi-
dential schools and orphanages between 1923 and 1940 was
around 8 percent. Taken together, these studies suggest that
about 6 percent of susceptibility to polio is due to close contact
with someone carrying the poliovirus, and about 30 percent is
due to your genes.

POLIO VIRGINS

Another line of evidence supports the power of genes in determining polio susceptibility. There have occurred a number of so-
called "virgin soil outbreaks," in which polio decimated
communities where no one had ever before been exposed to the
poliovirus and therefore no one had protective antibodies. In the
Canadian Arctic during the winter of 1948, an infected missionary
shared the poliovirus with a native Inuit community that had no
antibodies. Nearly half of the Inuit contracted polio, as compared
to 1 percent of all Canadians in 1948. Adults were the most

severely affected, and 25 percent of the Inuit died. Thirty-seven percent of the cases occurred in families, a percentage almost identical to the 36 percent in Herndon's identical twins, possibly due to Inuits living closely together combined with sharing genes due to intermarriage in their small, isolated community.

The Distaff Side of Polio

Another decidedly genetic factor that may be related to polio susceptibility is gender. Herndon found that more than 60 percent of the twins who got polio were male, while in Collins's national survey 40 percent more males than females had had polio. What's more, Collins found that 10 percent of males, versus 8 percent of females, died as a result of having polio, and 5 percent more males had lifelong paralysis. The poliovirus apparently likes boys best.

However, women may have been more at risk for polio at one time in their lives: during pregnancy. A twenty-year study of 325 women in Los Angeles found that those who were pregnant were twice as likely to get polio. Several smaller and shorter studies of more than 150 women found nearly three times more polio during pregnancy, although a lengthy Illinois study found no greater likelihood of polio in 400 pregnant women. Both the Los Angeles and Illinois studies found that polio and pregnancy was a dangerous combination. Pregnant women who developed polio were about five times more likely to die.

Overall, pregnant women seemed to have had about a 20 percent greater likelihood of getting polio, possibly because the hormonal changes that accompany pregnancy increase poliovirus susceptibility in some unknown way. Hormonal changes increasing susceptibility is also suggested by one study that found nearly 80 percent of women who got polio had had their menstrual period a few days before to a few days after the beginning of their illness.

Another question related to pregnancy was whether the fetus was at risk for getting polio from its infected mother. Of more than seven hundred pregnancies in women who had polio between 1934 and 1953, Los Angeles and Illinois obstetricians saw not one baby born with symptoms even vaguely similar to those of polio. Between 1897 and 1956, only seven cases were reported in medical journals of infants born with a paralyzed arm or leg, suggesting that the fetus had contracted polio many weeks before birth. It is likely that in these very rare cases, something unusual had happened. Perhaps the mother was not able to make enough poliovirus antibodies for herself and her baby, or her antibodies were not passed to the baby. Possibly some abnormality of the placenta allowed poliovirus to pass to the fetus. But overall, the chances of someone having caught polio inside the womb are "infinitesimal."

Genes and Other Means

So how is it that your genes made you more likely to get polio? There are several possibilities. Your genes may have made you less able to make enough poliovirus antibodies quickly enough to repel the poliovirus invasion. Your genes may have made your tonsils, intestines, Peyer's patches, and lymph nodes a more fertile breeding ground for the poliovirus. Your brain's blood vessels may have been more "leaky."

But the most likely genetic factor predisposing you to polio may be related to the poliovirus receptors. No matter how much poliovirus there is inside your body, it will have no effect without receptors on your neurons that are able to grab the virus and pull it inside. The remarkable thing about poliovirus receptors is that they also have a natural and important function within everyone's developing nervous system. In every four-month-old fetus, special proteins appear in the front of what will become the spinal cord and are evident all the way up through the center of the brain. These proteins send out signals that tell certain cells what they are to become when they grow up. Signaling proteins in the front of the spinal cord tell cells to grow into motor neurons; signaling proteins in the brain stem tell cells to become neurons that will activate the muscles of the throat, esophagus, diaphragm, and intestines. As the fetus develops, these signaling proteins disappear . . . almost. Like guests who have overstayed their welcome, some remain on the grown-up spinal cord and brain neurons and become a liability. Why? Because they have an unfortunate sideline: They can latch on to and unzip poliovirus. The remaining signaling proteins are the poliovirus receptors.

But the protein molecules that become poliovirus receptors may not remain on everyone's neurons. Back when David Bodian was trying to figure out how the poliovirus multiplied, entered, and damaged neurons, he intentionally infected monkeys with the virus. As few as 20 percent of monkeys that were fed large amounts of the most virulent strains of poliovirus by mouth, and only half of those whose muscles were injected with poliovirus, developed neuron damage as a result of poliovirus infection. So monkeys and humans who got polio may have a gene that allows lots of those signaling molecules to hang around after birth—and therefore have lots of poliovirus receptors. The more poliovirus receptors on your neurons, the more likely it is that they will be infected by even small amounts of poliovirus, and the more likely it is that your neurons will be damaged and you will become paralyzed.

INJURY AND POLIO

There is one means of increasing susceptibility to polio that has nothing to do with genetics: physical injury. For more than fifty years it has been known that children receiving intramuscular injections during a polio epidemic were up to ten times more likely to develop paralysis—paralysis that most frequently occurred in the limb where they'd received the injection. Injections break blood vessels and are thought to allow poliovirus-laden blood to bathe poliovirus receptors on motor nerves inside the muscles, which then take up the virus and allow it to enter the spinal cord.

Another type of injury is tonsillectomy, which actually exposed nerves in the throat to poliovirus growing there. Tonsillectomy was associated with the development of severe "bulbar" polio, since it's only a short trip from the throat to the brain stem.

Injury can also be caused by physical exertion. Exertion the day before polio symptoms became apparent has been associated with the development of paralysis; the more a given muscle was exercised, the more paralyzed it became. And exertion's ability to trigger or increase paralysis was more pronounced in adults. Of course, the best-known example of paralysis following exercise is the case of thirty-nine-year-old Franklin D. Roosevelt, who went swimming the day before his legs became severely paralyzed by polio.

Finally, emotional injury—stress—is known to suppress the immune system, causes the release of a variety of hormones, and has been suggested to increase susceptibility to all infections.

THE AGE EFFECT

A final "peculiar factor" related to polio susceptibility has to do with age, described in this Polio Paradox:

> **POLIO ATTACKED MOSTLY INFANTS EARLY IN THE TWENTIETH CENTURY. BUT INFANTS BECAME LESS AFFECTED AND TEENAGERS MORE AFFECTED AS THE DECADES WENT BY.**

Although the first outbreak of polio in any given year and any given location predominantly affected infants, each succeeding outbreak was less and less "infantile." In 1916, 80 percent of New York polio patients were less than four years old, a percentage that decreased to 50 percent in 1931 and to 20 percent in 1944. The disappearance of Infantile Paralysis also occurred after first epidemics in other parts of the country. In Massachusetts before 1916, nearly 70 percent of polio patients were less than four years old; by 1952 the number had dropped to less than 20 percent.

One reason Infantile Paralysis didn't remain primarily infantile may be related to mothers themselves. Once the poliovirus reached "critical mass" in a given densely populated area, it makes sense that those first affected in an epidemic would be infants—the one group in the community who'd certainly never experienced a polio outbreak before. Mothers were the group most likely to be exposed to poliovirus via their infected infants because they changed their babies' diapers. Since women in their twenties were highly unlikely themselves to be felled by polio, mothers may have developed antibodies and have been silent carriers of the poliovirus. Thus mothers may have infected other mothers with poliovirus, all of whom became natural vaccinators for future infants. The silent infection of large numbers of mothers and young children during an epidemic, causing widespread development of antibodies, explains in part why an epidemic in one year significantly decreased the chance of another polio epidemic in the following one or two years.

While mothers becoming natural vaccinators may in part explain the disappearance of Infantile Paralysis, it doesn't explain another aspect of the age effect: Polio patients were getting older as the decades went by. Although the percentage of five- to nine-year-olds who got polio was a relatively constant 30 percent from 1916 to 1954, the percentage of polio patients older than ten increased from less than 10 percent in 1916 to about 55 percent in 1952. Between 1950 and 1955, just over half of the polio patients admitted to one Massachusetts hospital were older than sixteen, and nearly a quarter were older than thirty. By 1955, 25 percent of polio patients were older than twenty.

Unfortunately, the older you were when you got polio, the worse its effects. Older polio patients had more limbs paralyzed, were paralyzed more severely, more frequently had chest and breathing muscle paralysis, and were three times more likely to die. Polio killed 3 percent of two-year-olds, 9 percent of ten-year-olds, and 20 percent of twenty-five-year-olds. Still, during the entire century the number of polio patients over twenty-five was at least thirteen times less than younger patients. This statistic makes sense of the fact that parents and the medical professionals treating polio survivors were unlikely to get polio.

Looking at the increasing age of polio patients, Albert Sabin could not understand why people did not become more immune to poliovirus infection as they aged, since older individuals had lived through many epidemics during which more and more people around them were getting polio. The older you were, the more opportunities you had to be exposed to poliovirus and develop antibodies. But immunity was not increasing as people aged during the middle of the twentieth century. Susceptibility actually increased, and survivability decreased.

To this day there is no clear explanation for the age effect. One possible explanation may have to do with the poliovirus itself. In monkeys the poliovirus can become more virulent—better able to enter and damage neurons—as it passes from animal to animal. Thus there seems to be a kind of natural selection process whereby virulent polioviruses become more dangerous as they move from host to host. The age effect may thus be due in part to poliovirus becoming more virulent as it passed from person to person from one year to the next. This process could explain poliovirus becoming more able to override older individuals' apparent natural resistance to polio as well as contribute to the nearly exponential increase in polio cases as the years went by.

The Polio Equation

By looking at all the factors that have been associated with polio, you can come up with a kind of equation to help understand why you may have contracted and been damaged by the poliovirus:

GENES

Having more poliovirus receptors, making fewer poliovirus antibodies,
or being a fertile ground for poliovirus multiplication

+

RACE

Being white, especially if you're of Germanic or southern European origin

+

BEING MALE

+

COMMUNITY EXPOSURE

Living in a congested city where there was lots of poliovirus, especially if
you had moved from a rural area and therefore had fewer antibodies

+

HOUSEHOLD EXPOSURE

Someone in your home had polio

+

POLIOVIRUS VIRULENCE

Being exposed to a powerful poliovirus

+

INJURY

Physical injury or overexertion, receiving an injection, or emotional stress

+

POLIOVIRUS "LOAD"

Being given a large dose of poliovirus

+

YEAR OF BIRTH

Being born later in the century

+

AGE

Having been an infant early in the twentieth century or a teenager in the
middle of the century

+

FEMALE HORMONES

Ovulating, just finishing a menstrual period, or being pregnant

---

POLIO

One Polio Survivor at a Time

Polio epidemiologist W. L. Aycock believed that epidemic polio
was in fact more common before 1890 than people realized. He
believed that there had been many "small" polio outbreaks, a few
handsful of cases scattered across the country. These outbreaks
might seem insignificant compared to the tens of thousands of
cases of polio each year during the 1950s. But ten cases of polio
in a town of a thousand people would be equivalent to ten thousand cases in a city of one million. To understand polio in a
country as big as the United States, Aycock suggested that you
need to think of any big polio epidemic as this sum of little outbreaks occurring in many individual cities or counties
throughout the country, caused by different types of polioviruses
with differing virulence, affecting different age and racial groups,
causing varying proportions of paralytic and "nonparalytic" polio.

I'll go one step farther. I think to understand polio—and especially to understand PPS—we need to think of the epidemics as
the sum of the varied effects of the poliovirus on everyone polio
touched. To do this, we need to understand not only the physical
but also the emotional damage done by polio, the effects that
damage had on polio survivors, their families, and society, both
immediately after poliovirus infection and for decades thereafter.

CHAPTER 5

"The Pest House"

New York Journal, August 25, 1916. Mrs. Jennie Dasnoit of 365 64th Street, Brooklyn, is under the care of a physician today as a result of a strange experience with the infantile paralysis quarantine. Three policemen forced their way into her home, broke down the door to her bedroom and drew their revolvers in assisting the ambulance surgeon to obtain possession of her small nephew, a paralysis suspect. The child, Cornelius Wilson, two-year-old son of Mrs. Dasnoit's dead sister, is in the Kingston Avenue Hospital, Brooklyn, where the physicians have not yet decided that he is suffering from paralysis. The policemen entered the house, Mrs. Dasnoit says, by cutting the screen covering a window on the first floor, breaking their way into the room where Mrs. Dasnoit stood with the baby in her arms. Stealing up behind her, they seized her arms. Their revolvers were drawn, she charges. Dasnoit's screams attracted neighbors to the house, but before they could enter two of the policemen held her while the third pulled the child from her arms and passed him through the window to the surgeon.

Polio was terror. Overwhelming, gut-wrenching terror. The terror generated by the first large American epidemic in 1916 caused people to do just about anything to escape The Dread

Disease. In New York, parents tried to pack their children onto trains and ferries to get them out of the infected city. But without a doctor's certificate proving absence of contagion, the children were turned back. When those with cars turned to the roads for escape, they were repelled by armed guards at the city limits.

Once escape from the city was made impossible, it was decided to contain the disease by isolating infected children within the city, as Mrs. Dasnoit discovered, whether families wanted their children "contained" or not. To house and treat the tens of thousands who contracted polio each year, special hospitals were built. And although the police were not typically employed to wrench polio survivors from their parents' arms, doctors and ambulance drivers ripping children suspected of having polio away from their families was wrenching enough.

The Initial Terror

I was taken from my parents without explanation, and wheeled into an elevator. That was when I came apart. I screamed all the way upstairs. A nurse wearing a mask over her nose and mouth hissed, Be quiet, you're only making it worse for everybody. But I was beyond terror.

MIA, CLASS OF '54

With the onset of symptoms, many polio survivors who understood that they had been stricken by The Dread Disease feared that disability was certain and death was likely. These fears were magnified in those who knew others who had been disabled or even killed by polio. Patients who come to The Post-Polio Institute describe the confusion, upheaval, and terror at being taken from their homes and being given by parents to strangers with whom they were required to live for weeks, months, or even years. Even children too young to understand what polio was certainly sensed their parents' fear and felt the desolation of being banished to polio hospitals.

In different parts of the country and during different decades, polio isolation hospitals were actually called "The Pest House." For some of our patients the Pest House was New York's Willard Parker Hospital. For many others the Pest House was an out-building, a former laundry, at the New York State Rehabilitation Hospital. This Pest House actually had bars on the windows:

> I had polio when I was five. I hadn't remembered a thing about the Pest House until I walked into Dr. Bruno's office. Then it all returned to me in a flash. I was taken 250 miles from home, admitted to the hospital, and didn't see my mother for two months. When I did see her again she was on one side of a glass window and I was on the other. She couldn't hold me, she couldn't comfort me. She couldn't even touch me.
>
> AUDREY, CLASS OF '43

Polio patients admitted to hospital quickly became aware of their complete loss of control and total dependence on the staff. Many patients could not feed or toilet themselves. Those with the most severe paralysis could not even move. Patients were forced to rely totally on hospital staff if their most basic needs were to be met. If they were to survive, patients had little choice but to suppress their fears and follow the instruction parents gave one of our patients as he was being taken from them: "Be good, don't make trouble, and do everything you're told so you'll get better."

PARADOXICAL PREDICTIONS

But *were* polio patients going to get better? Many tell the same story, sometimes verbatim, about their initial terrifying days in the hospital:

My parents were told that I might not make it through the night. Doctors kept an iron lung right outside the door to my room. Since I kept breathing and didn't need the iron lung, my parents were told I would live, but I was likely never to walk again. I was in the Pest House for a month and then moved up the hill to the rehabilitation hospital. I stayed there for over a year. I left the hospital on my own two feet, a brace on my right leg. So I did live and I did walk again in spite of what the doctors said. To this day my parents say my recovery was "a miracle."

ANNE, CLASS OF '51

Why would doctors tell parents on admission that their child might not live and then, within days, say that the child would likely not walk again? Did the doctors not know what they were talking about? Were they preparing parents for the worst or were they incompetent, even cruel?

Certainly the poliovirus could kill by damaging brain stem swallowing, breathing, and blood pressure control neurons and cause what was called "bulbar" polio. Although the numbers vary from year to year, as many as 15 percent of patients had "bulbar" polio. About a third of those had trouble breathing, either because their brain stem neurons stopped telling the diaphragm to move, or because the diaphragm and chest muscles themselves were paralyzed. Some who had trouble breathing needed the "iron lung," the long tanklike respirator in which your entire body, save your head, was placed and which "breathed" for you. About 70 percent of those in iron lungs died. Just over 50 percent with bulbar polio had trouble swallowing; 5 percent died. Almost 10 percent had trouble controlling their heart rate and blood pressure; over 80 percent died. So about one-third of "bulbar" polio patients did not make it.

All told, depending on the year and the city, less than 15 percent of polio patients died. Then why do so many of our patients remember their parents being told they wouldn't live through their first night in hospital? It's possible doctors were preparing parents for the worst-case scenario: That the child might develop bulbar symptoms even though he or she had none upon admission. It's possible that parents saw an iron lung in the hallway outside their child's room and assumed it would be necessary. But where else would an iron lung be but in the hallway near the rooms of those just admitted, at hand where it would have been immediately needed? So predictions of imminent death create another Polio Paradox:

MANY POLIO PATIENTS WERE TOLD THEY WOULD LIKELY DIE WHEN LESS THAN 15 PERCENT DID.

And what about doctors telling parents within days of the polio diagnosis that their child would never walk again? In the 1920s, when the numbers of those who had polio was relatively small and doctors' experience with long-term outcome was limited, it might have been reasonable to prepare parents for the worst, because doctors did not know what to expect. However, by the 1950s, statistics had been collected making it clear that the most likely outcome for anyone who had polio—even "bulbar" polio, even in some who had all four limbs initially paralyzed—was recovery to the point of partial paralysis of one lower leg. This presents another Polio Paradox:

POLIO PATIENTS WERE TOLD THEY WOULD NEVER WALK AGAIN WHEN ALMOST ALL DID.

I can't explain why doctors in the 1950s were telling parents that their children would never walk again. Again, it's possible doctors were preparing parents for the worst. But the unfortunate effect of dire predictions followed by "miraculous" recoveries was that polio survivors were set up for an even harder fall when they developed PPS and their abilities began to recede later in life.

The Long Road Back

When polio patients began to recover and muscles started working again, a long and painful road lay ahead, often beginning with a lengthy stay in a rehabilitation hospital. In the 1995 International Post-Polio Survey, we received questionnaires from more than eleven hundred polio survivors who told us about their polio and post-polio experiences. Ninety percent of those responding said they had been hospitalized after polio for an average of eight months. Hospitalizations in childhood could be devastating even to children who didn't have polio, especially back in the "dark ages" of medicine, as *Loneliness and Love* author C. E. Moustakas explains:

> Because of his inability to take care of himself in the all important functions, the possibility of being abandoned or left alone is the most serious threat to the child's whole existence. Of the many kinds of temporary abandonment, no experience is more desolating to a child than having to be in a hospital alone. The disrespect for the integrity of his wishes and interests, the absence of genuine human warmth, all enter into the loneliness of hospital life.

This description could have been written about polio patients, who entered the hospital with three strikes against them: They had been tainted by The Dread Disease, they had been torn away from their parents, and they were physically disabled. Polio hospital policies added even more desolation. Parents were actively kept away from their children. Parental visits, which one polio hospital nurse said "disrupted hospital routine and upset the children," were allowed rarely, briefly, or not at all. Brothers and sisters were typically never allowed to visit. Psychologist and polio survivor Mary Westbrook reports that at one hospital, parents were only allowed to call the switchboard operator during a certain hour, once a day, to receive a terse report on their child's condition: "good," "fairly good," or "serious." Nursing professor Lynne Dunphy states, "In many settings, families were allowed to visit only once a week. The idea was that complete separation from parents would help the children make a 'better adjustment' to their illness."

Patients discovered quickly that they were at the mercy of the staff, who used access to parents to control their young patients. The 1,185 polio survivors and 567 nondisabled individuals participating in our 1995 Survey were asked, among other things, to describe any experiences of emotional, physical, or sexual abuse:

> The nurse said, "Your parents are here and if you're good you'll be allowed to see them." My parents were never there because they were never allowed to come see me.

> Parents were allowed to visit only on Sunday from three o'clock to four o'clock. The nurses changed shift at three and gave report on the patients. They sat in the nurse's station and chatted and laughed and drank coffee while our parents waited at the front door and we all waited for them to be let in. On many Sundays the nurses let the parents in at three forty-five. My parents had to drive for over two hours just to get to the hospital.

> The nurses yelled at me when I cried after a visit from my mother and stopped her from visiting me again.

Three-quarters of polio survivors in our 1995 Survey told us that questions of hospital staff went unanswered or were not answered with concern:

> Although I was extremely upset and scared, no one would answer my questions about what was happening to me or explain why my parents couldn't come to see me.

> When I tried to ask a question the nurse cut me off, saying, "Every time you make a fuss you will have to stay here one day longer."

When the girl in the next bed asked a question the nurse slapped her and yelled, "I can't help it that you got polio!"

Recent research has shown that failing to answer questions of hospitalized young people, refusing to give even basic information—what had happened to them, what was going to be done to them and why—magnifies children's notions of the severity of their illness, often leading them to believe their illness is fatal, and they're likely to die.

There is no question that excellent and compassionate nursing care was given to many polio patients. But, especially at the height of the epidemics, some nurses were terrified that they would become infected, and most were overwhelmed by the sheer number of polio patients needing treatment. Overflowing wards provided assembly-line care as scores of polio patients were fed, bathed, and treated. Our 1995 Survey found that disruptions of this routine were neither tolerated nor accommodated:

> Just after I had polio I could not urinate. I couldn't go when the nurse wanted me to so I was beaten with a stick and dragged on the floor.

> Nurses made us wait and wait for a bedpan. Then they got nasty if we had an accident.

> Sometimes the nurses "forgot" to feed us. The nurses and aides slapped me, pulled my hair, and stuck me with needles if I complained.

Normal, childlike behaviors—tears or an angry word triggered by pain, fright, homesickness, even a nightmare—could result in extreme punishment:

> I had frequent nightmares and I would wake up crying. One nurse did not like my crying, especially because I sometimes would awaken the other patients. She came to

my bed and would say in a very threatening voice, "You stop crying or you are going to be sorry." One night I awoke crying from a nightmare. She came in and said, "I told you not to do this or you were going to be sorry." She pulled me in my hospital bed into a walk-in closet, turned off the light, closed and locked the door, and left me there until morning.

I made a picture on the wall with a crayon and was punished by being put in a laundry barrel and locked in a closet.

For three weeks I was confined to a straitjacket every night when I went to sleep. I still don't know what I did to deserve that.

Lynne Dunphy describes the ultimate in nurse's pique, control, and patient abuse:

I had a cloth around my neck to keep my neck from getting rubbed away by the collar [of the iron lung]. One day it slid . . . I couldn't breathe. I was crying and calling the nurse. You had to learn to really melt to get her attention. She came in and she seemed really frustrated, overworked, and just too busy. I told her what was wrong and she told me to stop crying. She said she would turn my respirator off if I didn't stop crying. When she did I passed out immediately.

Such anger and abuse from nurses was felt to be a very real threat to survival by patients who were isolated from parents and totally dependent on the staff. One patient described her hospital experience as being in constant "mortal danger."

"Physical Terrorists"

Actively ignoring polio patients' emotional and physical pain seems to have been part of the "therapeutic approach" to polio. In reviewing the publications of practitioners who treated polio during the epidemics, and polio survivors' biographies, Mary Westbrook found that there were two basic polio treatment "myths": First, that "contracting polio is not very upsetting for children. They soon get over their distress unless they are spoilt." Second, that polio patients should ignore their distress, since "hard work and cheerful acceptance overcome polio."

Application of these myths is evident in the actions of physical therapists who administered a daily regimen of painful and often frightening therapies. Through the early 1940s the treatment of choice for polio was limb immobilization to prevent muscles that weren't paralyzed from contracting and going into spasm, forcefully pulling a hand or foot in one direction and having it be permanently fixed in that position. Affected limbs were placed in casts or were bound in splints tied tightly onto legs and arms:

> The therapists tied splints to my legs and the nurses tied the splints to the bed. The gauze and straps cut into my skin. I would lie there in the morning calling out for hours until somebody came and took them off me.

> My splints were tied to the bed. When my birthday card fell on the floor I leaned over the side of the bed, couldn't get back up, and was hanging there by the straps. All thirty-five girls in the ward called for the nurse. She came in and yelled at me, humiliating me in front of all the other girls, and left me there, saying I would be paralyzed in that position forever.

When splints were removed, therapists forcefully pulled and pushed joints to move them to their normal position:

The physical therapist pushed up so hard on my foot that she broke the tendon in the back of my leg.

One physical therapist actually sat on my knee to stretch the muscles in my leg and I screamed and cried.

Once limbs had been straightened, tightly bound, heavy metal braces were applied to allow polio patients to stand on totally paralyzed legs and walk with the aid of crutches. Because walking with braces and crutches is so tenuous and frightening, therapists forced polio patients to stand and then pushed them down again so they could "learn how to fall without being hurt":

I guess physical therapists thought we'd be too frightened to try to stand up in our new braces. Some of the kids were. So therapists had these rubber truncheons, like short rubber nightsticks, and hit us until we'd stand up. Some would hit us if we fell down, even if they had pushed us down in order to teach us balance. When I protested this treatment I was told, "Jesus fell three times and he got up. Why should you complain?"

Another treatment, promoted by Franklin Roosevelt after his experience in the soothing warm springs at Pine Mountain, Georgia, was pool therapy. Warm water relaxed muscles, and its buoyancy reduced the pull of gravity, sometimes permitting weakened polio patients to stand. However, the physical benefits of a water therapy were sometimes outweighed by paralyzed patients' fears of being in the water:

I was always scared of water. I had never let my father teach me how to swim I was so scared. But we all had to have pool therapy. When I was in the hospital both my legs were paralyzed and my one arm was very weak. The therapist would put me on this board attached with chains to a crane, and push it out over the pool. The board would swing back and forth and I would scream and cry and cry

as she lowered me into the water. Every day I thought I was
going to drown.

Regardless of the treatment method, physical therapies were
often administered as if patients were on an assembly line,
without explanation, without parental consent, and certainly
without patients' consent. Young polio patients, isolated from
parents and totally dependent on staff, had no choice but to
allow therapists to do what they wanted, in spite of pain and fear.
In *The Long Road Back*, Larry Le Comte summarized polio
patients' relationships with therapists in his "unwritten hospital
rule": "Always tell them that you feel 'Better,' even if you know
you are dying."

"The Kenny Method"

As early as 1931, Henry and Florence Kendall of Baltimore's
Children's Hospital School recognized that immobilization with
splints and casts was preventing muscle contractions and joint
deformities but was not allowing muscles that still had functioning motor neurons to move again. The Kendalls recommended that initial splinting be followed by gentle massage of
muscle spasms, stretching, and careful muscle training.

But immobilization was still widely practiced in 1940 when a
self-taught nurse, Australian Elizabeth Kenny, came to America.
Kenny had a "new concept" of the cause and treatment of polio,
notions she said were "diametrically opposed to those accepted
throughout the medical world." It was Kenny's unshakable belief
that polio was a disease of the muscles, not the neurons, the
poliovirus causing muscles to go into spasm. During the spasm,
the motor neuron associated with the muscle could not function
and became inactive. When the spasm stopped, the muscle still
didn't move—not because the motor neuron was damaged, but
because it was "alienated" from its once-again-responsive
muscle. Kenny believed that polio paralysis was merely a form of

amnesia: Motor neurons had simply forgotten they were able to activate muscles.

Alienation did occur, possibly most often in polio patients who had been in casts and splints and had themselves "forgotten" to activate muscles that were immobilized and that they hadn't tried to move for weeks or months. Kenny's ability to identify polio patients whose muscles were alienated gave rise to the "Kenny Miracles," in which she was occasionally able to pluck paralyzed children from their beds and get them to walk.

Unfortunately, Kenny roiled at criticism of her alienation concept, ignoring contradictory evidence from polio researchers such as David Bodian, who proved that the poliovirus did indeed damage and kill motor neurons. It was this damage that caused muscles to go into spasm, either because of poliovirus damage to brain reticular formation neurons, or because the contraction of muscles whose motor neurons were less affected by the poliovirus was unopposed by muscles that had been paralyzed.

Kenny was equally dogmatic about the second half of her new concept of polio: treatment that rejected immobilization in favor of relaxing muscle spasm using her trademark hot "packs." Kenny demanded that only individuals she had trained—called "Kenny Technicians"—be allowed to practice what she wanted called "the Kenny method." A ninety-three-year-old registered nurse, trained during a six-month course by the Sister herself, wrote to me and described the Kenny method:

> Elizabeth Kenny did not use splints, casts, braces, or respirators. They were not needed, even for bulbar cases, if the patient had been treated properly. The first procedure Kenny advised was a cleansing enema. Every patient I saw started to improve after the enema, which flushed the remainder of the virus from the colon. After the enema, hot packs were started. Pack material was nearly pure wool, double thickness to prevent blistering, that would cover only the muscle and leave the joints free.

Packs were applied every two hours, kept on an hour and off an hour all day, with one covering the entire back when the patient was on their stomach. Packs were given more often in the acute stage and, with bulbar cases, sometimes every fifteen minutes. Packs were continued until full range of motion was achieved with no stiffness or contractions. Passive exercises and then active exercises were started as soon as tolerated. Therapy was continued until maximum recovery was reached, sometimes as much as five years.

One group of visiting doctors came to the ward where I was working and asked to receive a hot pack on his back. They are hotter than can be imagined, and he was furious. He said, "If my back blisters I'll sue."

The doctor's fury was understandable. The wool coming out of the boiling water was at 212 degrees Fahrenheit (100 degrees Celsius), so hot that therapists couldn't touch the packs with their hands:

Two times every day the therapists took hot packs out of the boiling water. The wool was too hot for them to touch so they used tongs. Every time they threw them on my bare legs I screamed.

The physical therapist took the hot pack out of the boiling water and pinned it to my hand so I couldn't pull away. My hand was badly burned and became infected.

Some of our patients and participants in the 1995 Survey report they still feel fear when they smell wet wool.

Kenny may not have known about Henry and Florence Kendall's successful massage and stretching protocol for polio, since she portrayed both her hot "packs" and muscle training method as "new." If Kenny had known, why would she have continued to advocate applying blistering heat that was not only unnecessary but dangerous? Said Florence Kendall:

Seldom discussed were the adverse reactions to the hot packs. An adult who was treated at age eight for polio says the heat treatments were the worst aspect of his illness, and to this day he cannot tolerate a hot bath. One boy was reported to have been hot-packed until his temperature reached 108 degrees F and he succumbed.

Some polio survivors responding to the 1995 Survey extolled Kenny's zeal, interest in children, and ability to motivate patients to try to move and walk. But some of her techniques to identify alienated muscles and her attempts to get polio patients to "take up their beds and walk" were painful, terrifying, and also dangerous:

Sister Kenny slapped me on the face several times as a means of "defining my reflex response."

Sister Kenny strode through the ward like General Patton, going from bed to bed examining each child, looking for something. When she got to my bed she apparently saw what she was looking for. She picked me up, put me under one arm, and walked down the hallway to the pool. She went to the side of the pool and threw me in, calling after me "sink or swim." My legs were totally paralyzed so I sank. Two therapists had to jump in to fish me out.

The story of the Kenny method reveals a double-edged sword that has implications for the treatment of PPS today. When the media and a 1946 film trumpeted the success of Kenny's mobilization of affected limbs, doctors were forced by public opinion to change their immobilization-only approach to the treatment of polio, very much as polio survivors today are forcing doctors to accept PPS and change their approach to the treatment of new fatigue, muscle weakness, and pain.

But Kenny's preeminence and her own dogmatism blotted out at least equally effective and more humane treatments for polio, such as the procedures developed by the Kendalls a decade earlier. What's more, Kenny relied not on scientific research but on testimonials from those who witnessed Kenny Miracles as proof of her "new concept" of polio, which was ultimately disproved. Polio survivors today need to be cautious of testimonials—even those of other polio survivors—promising treatments or cures or giving explanations for PPS that have not been scientifically tested.

MEDICAL MALPRACTICE

During the polio epidemics, nurses and therapists were far from being the only practitioners to cause polio patients physical and emotional pain. Doctors also were guilty of caring for, but not caring about, their patients:

> Doctors treated me like a subhuman slab of meat, a guinea pig, when I was twelve years old and in the hospital. A new group of doctors in training came to the polio ward every few months. On their first day I was stripped naked and left on a gurney in a room with the door open. Sometimes as long as an hour later, I would be rolled into a huge amphitheater filled with doctors in the white coats looking down at me. The head doctor would come in, sit me up, and say, "This is what polio looks like." He would turn me around so they could see the curve of my back, my scoliosis. He would force me to try to stand on my right leg that had no muscles. The tears would just roll down my face but I didn't make a sound. I knew what the nurses would do to me if I made a fuss.

> While I was asleep one night the doctor came to draw blood from an artery in my groin. I woke up when the needle stuck me and a fountain of blood was squirting toward the ceiling. They left me soaked in my own blood until morning.

I had been in an iron lung for weeks. There was a doctor who kept taking me out of the iron lung before I could breathe on my own. Every time he took me out I turned blue. He did this over and over again, forty or fifty times. I was three years old.

Overt thoughtlessness and abuse on the part of some physicians may have resulted from their being unable to cure polio. Polio survivor Charles Mee wrote that doctors were "mostly irrelevant and they knew it. Some doctors must have been embarrassed by this, or angry, maybe." Given the circumstances, physicians expected at the very least not to be troubled by their incurable charges. Regina Woods recalls physicians insisting "that I be only what they want me to be, an easily pliable 'patient' who asks no questions."

A DISTAFF SIDE TO ABUSE

Our 1995 Survey also found that polio patients were not only emotionally and physically abused, but also sexually abused. Sexual abuse was most common among female polio patients and was perpetrated by staff members at all levels, from physicians to orderlies. Many polio patients who were abused—especially those who were sexually abused—said nothing about it, not even to their parents:

The doctor was supposed to be able to do whatever he wanted to me. I allowed him to abuse me because I would have made my parents angry if I was not doing what I was told. And I was afraid the nurses, who I depended on for everything, would have punished me for making trouble. All I could do was stop feeling bad about what he did to me and smile.

I was always told how independent and strong I was. My mother told everyone, "My girl doesn't get homesick or cry."

Why cry about what the orderlies were doing to me at night, to make my parents feel guilty? They were not going to let me come home if I cried and I didn't want to disappoint them. They needed to believe that I was okay so I put on a brave face. I never told anyone about the abuse . . . ever.

Female polio patients were abused in another way. Many were told by doctors that they could never, should never, would never have a child. There were typically no medical reasons for this prohibition, either on the basis of polio patients' physical condition or the medical literature on pregnancy after polio:

> I was in the hospital for just a few months when I was ten. My only disability was that my foot was paralyzed and I wore a short leg brace. My orthopedic doctor, my gynecologist—even my family doctor—told me I would never survive a pregnancy and, if I did, I would never have a "normal" child. I wanted to prove them wrong so I had five healthy children.

For some female polio patients, pregnancy was not even an issue, since hospital staff made it clear that they would never date or marry, let alone have sex and become pregnant. Polio patients were often told that they were ugly, unlovable, and incompetent, that they would find neither a job nor a mate:

> We had a tutor in the hospital. She always looked angry and frightened. We thought she was worried we would give her polio. I was very good in school and when I did well on a test she got angry at me. After I had gotten 100 on a spelling test, she said to me, "That's all right. No one is ever going to give you a job anyway."

Almost 15 percent of polio survivors responding to our 1995 Survey were emotionally, physically, or sexually abused in the hospital. Moreover, nearly one-third were abused in more than one way and 60 percent were abused more than once, from twice, to weekly, to daily, to "too many times to count." Emotional, physical, and sexual abuse in the hospital were more common in our Survey in those who were younger when they had polio, had polio during the late 1940s and 1950s, were more disabled, and especially if they were girls.

GO ALONG TO GET ALONG

Isolation from family, along with neglect and abuse by those who held polio patients' lives in their hands, made it clear that survival depended upon suppressing needs and emotions and unquestioningly complying with those in authority. A group of Baltimore psychiatric researchers studying hospitalized polio survivors described them as "good patients," some of whom accepted "immobilization and other forms of restraint and inactivation with a certain contentment and submission." Their observation of "contentment and submission" is reminiscent of "The Stockholm Syndrome," in which hostages ally with their captors and even join in their cause. Some patients at Baltimore's City Hospital during the 1950s submitted so completely to the hospital staff that they did not wish to go home or even asked to be returned to the hospital when they were discharged. Some polio patients overidentified with the staff, wanting to become orthopedic surgeons and nurses when they grew up. But other polio patients were already practicing as nurses. Polio patients fed other children who were unable to feed themselves and bottle-fed babies on the infant polio wards. Those who were older when they were hospitalized and who had regained some function started caring for "new recruits" who were less able:

> We would watch out for each other. When someone was going to surgery the next morning, especially if it was their first surgery, those of us who had been "upstairs" would explain what it was like, what to expect before and after.

When they came back down from the recovery room we would sit by the bed and hold their hands.

One older boy made it his business to make sure that every other child on his ward was safe:

I would wheel over to each of them before I went to bed. One boy caught pneumonia. The nurses seemed not to notice so I kept telling them he was getting sicker and sicker. Finally the doctor was called and they put him in an oxygen tent. After lights-out I got back in my wheelchair and went to his bed. His lips were blue and he couldn't talk so I just held his hand. I woke up as a nurse pulled my hand away from his. He had died sometime during the night.

Under these circumstances, some polio survivors lost their own identities:

I was seven years old when I went to the hospital. For two weeks I didn't know who I was. I asked every person who went by, "Who am I? What's my name?"

If you get hit for whining or crying you get tough. I found I got by by having a positive attitude. I did what I thought was best for me: Don't complain, keep your true feelings to yourself, make jokes about your disability so other people will be more at ease and accept you, be tough and never, never cry. It turns out this probably wasn't the best way to be because I lost myself. I'm not sure who the real me is. I'm not sure I want to even know the real me.

In a desperate effort to protect himself and hold on to his identity, one polio survivor stopped speaking in the hospital and physically tried to fight off attempts by doctors, nurses, and therapists to treat or even touch him. He refused to have his hair cut or speak for the year he was hospitalized.

Certainly, some polio survivors have pleasant memories of

being in the hospital, of staff members who cared for them and even showed them unusual kindness. There were wheelchair races and toys contributed by local organizations. Volunteers would visit the polio wards, play games, and hold special parties. But at best, said one polio survivor, "We were cared for but we weren't cared about or nurtured or loved."

So polio survivors learned to deal with their abandonment, loss of control, fear, pain, and abuse by submitting to those in authority, complying fully with staff expectations, denying personal needs as well as physical and emotional pain—sometimes even denying their own individuality. This resignation to authority can be seen in items from the "Good Chart" written by polio ward mates at Baltimore's City Hospital:

LISTEN TO THE DOCTORS

OBEY THE NURSES

DO NOT FIGHT

BE A GOOD SPORT

DO NOT BE BAD

BE GOOD IN SCHOOL

DO YOUR HOMEWORK

DO NOT TALK AT DINNER, AT NIGHT OR IN SCHOOL

LITTLE FOLKS SHOULD BE SEEN AND NOT HEARD

When polio patients returned home, the "Good Chart" became their prescription for proper behavior. They had learned very young and very well that submission, compliance, and suppression of emotion were required if they were to escape the "mortal danger" that was polio.

CHAPTER 6

You Can't Go Home Again

The front yard is my playground, my world—no, my universe! My universe: my ten- by fifteen-foot front yard. This is where I ride my bike, where I play, where I spend my days. I'm an only child, pampered, spoiled, and protected by my parents. My mom and dad will not allow me to leave the yard but have given me all the toys, all the latest gadgets: Fort Apache, Lionel trains, battalions of army men. Mom says, "Your cousins and the other kids on the block will come to play with you." But no one comes. They're all in the schoolyard having fun. Mom bribes them to keep me company and they come for my toys, not for me. When they come to my front yard, they come for the freak show. There is no admission charge to play with the freak. And after you play for a while you can hit the freak in the head with a baseball bat or steal some of his toys. The freak has so many toys no one will notice.

Sunday nights I am really anxious. Tomorrow I go to school. It's scary outside my little universe. In school I'm a loner. If I walk real fast and don't look up no one will see me, no one will see my limp. Every Monday is Blue Monday.

Anxiety, inferiority, uselessness. Fear in the pit of my stomach is always there, for as long as I can remember. It is haunting me. Why? I had polio. That's why.

JAMES, CLASS OF '49

When polio survivors left the hospital and reentered their communities, the abuse didn't stop. It sometimes became worse.

The Sorrow and the Pity

Polio survivors entered the real world that was itself disabled by polio in many ways: Children were isolated in their homes during epidemics, theaters and pools closed to stop the spread of contagion. Terror was triggered by every summer cold and fever.

Capitalizing on America's fear of polio, in 1946 the National Foundation for Infantile Paralysis began its infamous campaign using pictures of children disabled by polio to raise money. The March of Dimes "poster children" were shown in wheelchairs or clad in heavy metal braces, leaning tenuously on their crutches. They called down from their posters to America's mothers and fathers, asking them to give money to help find a polio vaccine. One billboard showed a little girl in a big wheelchair, brace on one leg and dolly on her lap, looking out accusingly, with the caption, I COULD BE YOUR CHILD.

> My parents rarely said no when the March of Dimes asked to use me to raise money since they paid for my therapy. I knew just what to do, on television or when they were taking pictures: where to look and especially how to look sad. They always asked me to look sad. The most upsetting experience was when they put me up on a table, wearing my brace and with crutches, and took pictures as I watched my brother and sister cry as they got their polio vaccine shots.
>
> MOIRA, CLASS OF '52

The March of Dimes poster children created another Polio Paradox:

**THE VERY CAMPAIGN THAT RAISED MONEY TO PAY FOR
POLIO SURVIVORS' THERAPIES AND EQUIPMENT CAUSED
THEM TO BECOME SOCIAL PARIAHS.**

The posters were everywhere, ubiquitous reminders of the terror that was polio. When polio survivors returned home, it was not uncommon for them to discover that their entire family had been shunned because they had all been tainted by The Dread Disease. Said one polio survivor, "My having polio caused the complete isolation of my family by our entire small town. My family was shunned and hated by everyone."

Friends, sometimes even relatives, afraid of contagion or unable to deal with polio striking so close to home, severed ties with "afflicted" families. People crossed the street to avoid walking in front of a home where someone was known to have had polio. Many avoided contact with "polio victims" for fear that the "crippling" was contagious. Polio survivors told us about their experiences in the 1995 Survey:

> Years after I had polio, when adults saw me coming they would say out loud to their children to stay away from me because they could "catch it." My brothers and sisters did not want my "bad leg" to touch them.

Polio survivors' braces and crutches were repulsive reminders of everyone's vulnerability to the poliovirus:

> A stranger accosted me on the street and accused me of "upsetting people," saying, "You cripples shouldn't be allowed in public!"

Polio survivor J. B. Emory described the shame of having polio, writing that admitting he'd had "infantile paralysis was beyond me. I would more readily have told them I had leprosy." Polio survivors felt unclean, unwanted, and isolated. Polio survivors were the AIDS children of their generation.

Sticks and Stones

Without a doubt the worst offenders in terms of emotional and physical abuse when polio survivors returned home were their own peers. Children can be very cruel to those who are different. The slow, hobbling, clanking leather-and-steel-clad polio child could not have been a more inviting target for abuse:

> I had almost no balance when I stood on my crutches. Boys would run by me in the hall and knock me down. I was chased and hit. The other boys threw stones at me. It was a game for them.

> Every morning I put on my leg braces, took my crutches, and walked a mile to school. When I got to the building the boys were waiting for me at the top of a long flight of stone stairs. They would yell and throw garbage at me during the fifteen minutes it took to climb those stairs.

In addition to sticks and stones, names were also hurled at polio survivors:

> *Ugly, lazy, hateful, dumb,*
> *Peg-leg, iron legs, little foot, gimp,*
> *Cripple, limpy, gimpy, slow poke,*
> *Clumsy, klutz, retarded reject,*
> *Worthless, useless, bone-arm . . . Polio Boy.*

I was deeply sensitive about my condition and used many a stratagem to conceal my weakness. The severest crisis, however, came when my own generation started snickering. That was a time when boys in their early teens wore knee britches and black stockings. One day as I was en route to school . . . a group of boys my age caught up with me. One of them, whom I did not know, commented jeeringly, "Look at that kid's skinny legs. Aren't they something? Did you ever see anything as funny?" The others laughed; then a boy said, "I sure would cover them up if they were mine."

The words were like a lash across my face. I was depressed for weeks and months after that episode. I was humiliated and ashamed. I wanted to quit school to go into hiding. I became a semi-recluse, staying indoors as much as possible.

Justice William O. Douglas, Class of '01

Even when polio survivors were allowed to play with neighborhood children or former friends, they often couldn't keep up because of weak muscles, braces, and crutches. Polio survivors were further isolated from society because they were no longer physically able to participate easily or fully in social activities:

The others mimicked me, the way I walked. I was never chosen to play games with other children, I was never picked for sports teams. I was completely alone.

Parents: Absent, Guilty, and Abusive

When many polio survivors returned home from the hospital, they were eagerly received by their parents. Some parents completely dedicated themselves to their children, providing compassionate and appropriate care, both emotional and physical. For some no amount of expense, time, or effort was too great to help their child recover:

My brother Thomas and I had polio at the same time, when I was nine and he was eleven. When I returned home from Cook County Hospital, the Sister Kenny treatment was started immediately. We spent the entire day, from morning till late at night, wrapped in hot wet wool and heavy plastic. Curiously the disease brought the two of us and all of the family close together.

EDWARD CARDINAL EGAN, CLASS OF '42

Unfortunately, some polio survivors' families were riven by polio:

I had polio when I was four. My parents admitted me to the hospital and never came back to visit. When I was twenty-two the polio epidemics were over and the hospital was closing. I had to leave the hospital. I haven't seen my parents to this day.

H. A. Robinson and a team of mental health researchers at a Baltimore children's hospital concluded that many polio patients developed a "pervasive feeling of guilt," believing that polio, rejection, and abuse were deserved punishments, thinking "a terrible thing has happened to me—I must have done something terrible to make it happen." Some polio survivors report that they do feel guilty, as if they had done something for which polio was an appropriate punishment:

The day before I got polio I hit my friend in the leg. When my leg became paralyzed I thought God was punishing me and my leg for hurting my friend.

Polio researcher Sol Rosenbaum also reported that guilt was a typical response of parents to their child's polio: When polio was first diagnosed, "parents will almost certainly ask themselves, 'Why did this happen to us? What is it that we have done, or have failed to do to make this terrible thing possible? Just where have we failed our child?'" Rosenbaum also believed that parents thought, albeit unconsciously, "Since we can discover no willful neglect on our part, isn't it possible that this is somehow the child's fault?"

In addition to guilt, Rosenbaum noted that parents developed "resentment at the loss of freedom to continue their accustomed ways of living, and the feeling that somehow they have been greatly wronged." Polio survivors describe parents who were angry as if it were they, and not their child, who had been attacked by polio:

> When polio struck I was totally paralyzed and my mother screamed into my face, "Why are you doing this to me?" Mother blamed me for family problems even when they really had nothing to do with my polio.

> My mother complained about how expensive my braces were, how much she had to give up to care for me. She would fly into a rage and begin beating and slapping me. She once grabbed the bottom of my braces and pulled my feet out from under me. I hit my head on the sink as I fell.

> My father beat me all the time, telling me I was worthless, that he wished I'd never been born, that he wished the polio had killed me.

> When I just had polio my father and sister would slap me, kick me, and yell at me, telling me I was no good. They would take my things away from me and put them just out of reach. When I got older, my father expected me to pull my own weight on the farm. He slapped me because I couldn't do the work he wanted me to do.

Some parents were desperate to remove the stigma of disability and the responsibility of caring for a "helpless cripple":

> My father would hit me if he saw me using my wheelchair instead of my crutches.

> My father said that he would rather see me "dead than a cripple." He would make me take off my braces in the kitchen and try to stand up and walk without even my crutches. I would somehow get up and then fall down.

When I fell he would hit my head against the refrigerator and make me stand again. One day he got so frustrated that I couldn't walk he threw me down the cellar stairs.

And when polio survivors refused to be cured by their parents' "ministrations," one alternative to acceptance was internal exile or imprisonment. Some polio survivors report being physically trapped by their parents' refusal to make accommodations for their physical limitations. Homes frequently remained inaccessible, making activities of daily living impossible without assistance from parents—assistance that could be inconsistently provided or consistently withheld:

I was in the hospital for thirteen months and was in a wheelchair the entire time. It was no surprise to my parents that I wasn't going to be walking when I came home. Yet they never put a ramp into the house. My bedroom and our only bathroom were on the second floor. I had polio when I was six and until the day I moved out of the house to go to college not one accessibility modification had been made.

My mother beat me, but that wasn't the worst. She went to work at 7:30 A.M. and put me out on the front porch in my wheelchair, rain or shine, summer or winter. I was brought inside when she came home.

For almost two years after I got out of the hospital, I lived in an upstairs room of the house. My mother never let me out once until I was nineteen and was able to arrange to leave on my own.

My parents would just leave me in bed for hours staring at the ceiling. Sometimes they wouldn't even bring me food. I felt abandoned, unloved, unworthy, betrayed . . . and for some reason guilty. I was suicidal as a teenager and filled with anger and rage as an adult.

Nearly 40 percent of polio survivors in our 1995 Survey reported that they were emotionally, physically, or sexually abused at home. Of these, three-quarters were abused in more than one way, and nearly 80 percent were abused more than one time— from twice to weekly, to daily, to abuse that was said to be "ongoing" or "constant."

Amnesia and Expectations as Abuse

Some parents strove to reincorporate their child into the family routine and to "forget" about polio by requiring children to equal or exceed their level of physical activity before the illness:

All of a sudden my family took up hiking when I came home from the hospital, expecting me to "keep up with the others" in spite of my crutches and braces.

My mother constantly demanded that I be *normal*. I was an embarrassment to her and her family. I was the "odd note." My disabilities were covered up and I was always supposed to be better than everyone else.

If polio survivors couldn't outperform peers physically, they were expected to outperform academically, and do it with a smile:

I was always expected to be cheerful and not show real emotions. I would be severely punished if I received anything less than an A.

I always had to be better than everyone else, all grown up. I was never to cry even when I was spanked.

I couldn't complain or feel sorry for myself. Handicapped people shouldn't do those things because they're expected of us. Above all I must not fail!

I struggled valiantly to be as much like, or better than— especially better than—every other child in every other way that I could. Since I couldn't compete physically, I would be smarter. And indeed, I started first grade a year early and skipped fifth grade and earned excellent grades. I also earned respect from my elders and, because I was always ahead of my age group, was further isolated from my contemporaries.

The idea that I was a weakling festered and grew in my mind. I decided to prove my superiority over my contemporaries in other ways. Even a boy with weak and puny legs can get straight A's, I said to myself. No one would excel me in school. So I threw myself into that endeavor, and came very close to making the perfect scholastic record which I had set as a goal.

JUSTICE WILLIAM O. DOUGLAS, CLASS OF '01

Sol Rosenbaum described "Mary," the ideally adapted polio survivor, a "lively, happy child with a well-rounded personality":

Kindergarten was a happy experience for Mary and, as though in compensation for her handicap, she excelled in many things which required purely mental prowess. She had learned by this time to protect herself against other children, for in their thoughtless preoccupation in play they would frequently knock her down, sometimes painfully. But Mary would laboriously pick herself up, spurning all assistance, and rejoin the play activities without resentment or malice toward the offenders.

Author Bentz Plagemann, a polio survivor himself, provided in his 1955 novel *This Is Goggle* a model for appropriate post-polio behavior:

Jeanie Benson was a pretty little girl, with soft, dark hair and a direct, rather impudent way of looking at you. But more than beauty, Jeanie had courage. She was a victim of polio. She wore braces on her legs, as she walked to school from her house one block away on crutches.

With her shining face and shining crutches she made her entrance into the lunchroom. Jeanie's secret was that she knew how to laugh at her predicament. Everything amused her: her difficulty with walking, the troublesome knee locks on her braces, which sometimes did not unlock when she sat down, so her legs stuck straight out in front of her like the legs of a wooden doll, and reduced her and everyone around her to hysteria. She laughed at her awkwardness at getting up or down stairs, and, when she became exhausted and had to stop, a little, intimate world sprang into being around her. She possessed that wonderful faculty of making everything entertaining.

Difficulty walking, troublesome knee locks, awkwardness, and exhaustion. Yes, that's entertainment.

Be "all grown up," excel in school, ignore physical abuse and pain, suppress emotions, reject assistance, and make everybody happy. Be "normal"? No, be better than everyone else. Polio survivors' behavior when they returned home was an echo of the hospital's "Good Chart," motivated by a denial of polio and revulsion at their disability. The expectations of academic performance and suppression of emotion reinforced the stoic and adult behaviors learned in the hospital, causing polio survivors to grow up far too soon. As Mia Farrow writes in the first line of her autobiography, "I was nine when my childhood ended." Mia was nine when she got polio.

As polio survivors left childhood behind, many replaced their own sense of self with the powerful expectations of nurses, therapists, doctors, and parents—of society itself—that dictated the behaviors that were required if polio survivors were to escape "mortal danger." Polio survivors continued to follow the prescription for "proper" behavior set forth in the "Good Chart" in order to be tolerated, to prevent abuse—even possibly to be accepted—but at the very least to survive.

CHAPTER 7

Becoming "Normal"

I'll walk without crutches. I'll walk into a room without scaring everybody half to death. I'll stand easily enough in front of people so that they'll forget I'm a cripple.

FRANKLIN D. ROOSEVELT, CLASS OF '21

Where Is That Little Girl?
She is sick, her family is concerned.
Where is that little girl?
She's been taken apart and put together again by the
    surgeons.
Like a fledgling about to leave the nest for the first time
She is testing the waters of a normal life.
Can she catch up? Can she achieve? Can she excel?
Certainly, she must.

RUTH MIHALENKO, CLASS OF '39

Polio survivors were left with baggage that was too heavy for any child—or teenager, or adult—to bear:

- The terror and taint of having The Dread Disease.
- The fear and then reality of physical disability.

- Isolation from parents, family, and community.
- Hospitalization and dependency.
- The pain of physical therapy and surgeries.
- Submission to authority and denying personal needs and feelings.
- Emotional, physical, and sexual abuse.

What did polio survivors learn from their experience of fear, pain, abuse, and rejection? Polio survivors learned from parents, family, teachers, friends—that to be even marginally accepted back into society, they must become "normal."

Physical Normalcy

If polio survivors were to function in a totally inaccessible world, even paraplegic polio survivors learned that they must maximize whatever physical abilities remained and be able to get up and walk.

> I was ten years old when I left the hospital. My legs hadn't moved since I was five and I had worn two full-length leg braces. But the doctors told me when I was discharged, "You'll walk out of those braces before your senior prom."
>
> JANET, CLASS OF '54

Such calls to normalcy embodied not one Polio Paradox but two:

WHEREAS POLIO PATIENTS WERE TOLD ON ADMISSION TO THE HOSPITAL THAT THEY WOULD DIE OR NEVER WALK AGAIN, ON DISCHARGE THEY WERE GIVEN THE PROMISE OF FULL RECOVERY.

**THE BRACES, CRUTCHES, AND WHEELCHAIRS THAT HAD
MADE MOBILITY POSSIBLE, THAT HAD BEEN SYMBOLS OF TRI-
UMPH OVER PARALYSIS IN THE HOSPITAL, AT HOME BECAME
STIGMATA OF THE DREAD DISEASE.**

Assistive devices also became symbols of doctors'—and polio
survivors'—failure to have conquered polio. This notion of
failure was shared by the general public and amplified by the
development of the polio vaccine in 1954. Contributions to the
March of Dimes dropped after 1954. At least to those no longer
threatened by the possibility of paralysis, polio "had ceased to
be a vital concern," according to Jane Smith, author of
Patenting the Sun, a history of the Salk polio vaccine. Americans appeared to believe that the vaccine was actually a cure
for polio: "It seemed that the public expected the past victims
of polio to rise up and walk away, cured by the miracle" of the
vaccine, wrote Smith. "Once lionized as heroic examples of
human fortitude, the thousands of polio survivors who continued to need medical attention and financial help were suddenly ignored as embarrassing emblems of their own poor
timing, clumsy enough to get polio before the vaccine that
could have protected them was found."

Polio survivors did indeed try to "rise up and walk away,"
working to discard assistive devices regardless of weakness,
fatigue, and the constant danger of falling as they strove for the
appearance of complete physical normalcy. Painful and
exhausting physical therapies were resumed upon patients'
return home from the hospital or initiated in those who were not
hospitalized. Physical therapy often continued for more than a
decade after the polio attack, with the only acceptable goal being
a complete "cure":

My right leg and left arm had been paralyzed and I had
always used a wheelchair. I came home from the hospital
when I was seven and started physical therapy all over
again. I continued daily physical therapy with my mother,
went to the PT every week, until I left home for college.

Everyone—including me—believed that physical therapy would make me walk . . . eventually.

NANCY, CLASS OF '49

In 1955 pioneering British polio researcher W. J. W. Sharrard reported results of a three-year study of his polio patients. He found that there was "little further benefit" from physical therapy continuing more than ten months after the polio attack. Then why did polio survivors in our 1995 Survey report that they had an average of thirty-three months of physical therapy? To become "normal," of course. Over the years, through Herculean effort and an uncanny ability to substitute working muscles for those that were weak or paralyzed, many polio survivors were able to discard wheelchairs, braces, and crutches. Both S. D. Collins's survey and our Post-Polio Surveys showed that the typical polio patient had both legs affected initially but was able to walk at the peak of his or her recovery with at most a short leg brace. So the overwhelming majority of polio survivors were able to walk without stigmata of The Dread Disease, regardless of how tenuous, ungainly, painful, and frightening it was to walk. Polio survivors could become "normal." It is understandable that one-quarter of the polio survivors in the 1985 Survey told us they did not think of themselves as having a disability before developing PPS. They had been "cured."

The Unkindest Cut

In many polio survivors, motor neurons did not recover, and muscles did not regain sufficient strength through physical therapy alone to allow walking without assistive devices. For those polio survivors one hope of normalcy remained: the surgeon's knife. As far back as the 1830s, American orthopedic surgeons were performing operations on polio survivors. One-fifth of survivors in our 1995 Survey reported having been hospitalized after polio for an average of six months for a variety of orthopedic surgeries.

NIPPING, TUCKING, AND STAPLING

A number of procedures were performed to rid polio survivors of braces and crutches and to get them on their feet. The most common were tendon lengthenings, ankle fusions, and bone staplings. A polio survivor told us in chapter 5, "The physical therapist pushed up so hard on my foot that she broke the tendon in the back of my leg." In many polio survivors the Achilles tendon in the back of the leg became shortened when the anterior tibialis muscle, the muscle in the front of the leg that pulls the foot upward, became paralyzed. This was the muscle most commonly affected by the poliovirus and caused the "withered limb and dropped foot" that tells us that the Egyptian priest Rom had polio. The heel of a foot with a shortened Achilles tendon can't be placed flat on the ground. So the Achilles tendon, also called the "heel cord," was cut and lengthened. If the muscle had been totally paralyzed, the ankle was also fused by tucking pieces of bone into the joint to stop the foot from dropping down. These procedures allowed polio survivors with a paralyzed lower leg to walk without using a short leg brace.

Another surgery performed to allow polio survivors to discard braces was the muscle transplant—moving a working muscle from one side of the foot or knee to do the job of a muscle that was paralyzed on the other. In this way someone with a partially paralyzed quadriceps, the muscle in the front of their upper leg, could again "lock" their knee and stand without a long leg brace.

Another common operation was the placement of metal staples in the growth plate of the femur, the thigh bone, on the side that was less affected by polio. The leg with paralyzed muscles was usually shorter than the less affected leg, probably because there were no muscles pulling on the bone—pulling causing calcium to deposit and allowing the bone to grow. The less affected leg was stapled to stop its growth, thus preventing the legs from being different lengths and eliminating the need for a large and unsightly buildup on the sole of one shoe.

TWISTS AND TURNS

The pulling of functioning muscles, unopposed by muscles that had been paralyzed, sometimes resulted in joint deformities despite casting and splinting. Sometimes, if the lower leg and foot twisted to the right or left, an osteotomy was performed: The tibia, the lower leg bone, was cut in two, turned, and set so that the foot pointed forward.

The lack of muscles pulling evenly on both sides of the spine caused scoliosis—a C- or S-shaped side-to-side curvature of the back—in about a third of polio survivors. If the curve was severe enough, a spinal fusion was performed, using chips of bone cut from the hip to lock the vertebrae together and straighten the spine:

> I knew that someday the doctor would come up with an operation my mother couldn't refuse. She finally agreed to a spinal fusion. It was done in two steps. First I was fused from my neck to the middle of my back. A few days later I was fused the rest of the way. I lay unmoving in my parents' living room in a chin-to-knees body cast for six months.
>
> NANCY, CLASS OF '49

If these extreme procedures failed to achieve normalcy, more unorthodox surgical options were available. In one especially brutal procedure, available briefly in the 1940s, an electric rivet gun was used to pulverize paralyzed muscles and their motor nerves "into a mass of jelly" to encourage axons to sprout—a uniquely medieval attempt to increase muscle strength and prevent the need for assistive devices.

ABUSE REDUX

Whatever the procedure, polio survivors were again ripped away from families, hospitalized, and forced to endure the new fears and pain associated with surgery and anesthesia. What's worse, some survivors had not one but as many as a dozen separate procedures over the years to straighten, strengthen, stabilize, and normalize their bodies:

> Almost every summer from the time I was two years old I would have another operation. No one would tell you what they were going to do. The night before and the morning of surgery were the worst. The night before you got an enema and were shaved—embarrassing. They promised you a balloon if you were good. *Big deal!* In the operating room I would pretend that the ether was working and then try to rip the mask off my face and get away. I knew the ether would make me throw up later for hours. When I did wake I was in pain and nauseous. No child should have to live through that even once!
>
> MOIRA, CLASS OF '52

Surgery added even more emotional insults to additional physical injury. Participants in our 1995 Survey who were hospitalized for surgery had an increased likelihood of being emotionally and physically abused. And those polio survivors who needed surgery were *already* more likely to have been emotionally, physically, and sexually abused, since they were more physically disabled and therefore easier targets.

A Post-Polio Personality?

Whether they were hospitalized or treated at home; significantly recovered, surgically rebuilt, or forever braced; overtly or covertly abused—the polio experience was unlikely to have left polio survivors unscathed. But what was the emotional fallout of having been touched by The Dread Disease?

When polio survivors first came to us twenty years ago reporting new symptoms, I didn't consider that there were psychological consequences of having had polio, let alone that there were psychological aspects of PPS. However, the first three polio survivor subjects in our first study in 1983 made it clear that something unusual was happening not only below but also above the neck. All three used power wheelchairs. The first, a federal official with a graduate degree, had one arm and leg paralyzed; the next was quadriplegic and the director of the New York City mayor's Office on the Disabled; the third, also quadriplegic, was the chief executive officer of a New York corporation. As I continued to work with polio survivors, I realized that they all seemed to be cut from the same cloth. Regardless of their disabilities, these individuals were at least college graduates and had risen to high levels—if not the highest level—of their chosen professions. I met polio survivors who were corporate CEOs, executive vice presidents, and professionals of all types—teachers, lawyers, doctors. No polio survivor was unemployed. These polio survivors point out a startling Polio Paradox:

POLIO SURVIVORS WHO WERE TOLD THEY WOULD NEVER GO TO COLLEGE OR GET A JOB BECAME THE COUNTRY'S BEST AND BRIGHTEST.

Polio survivors were obviously unique, not only among individuals who had disabilities of equal severity, but also among their nondisabled peers of similar age. It appeared that our patients shared a personality type that had first been described among those at risk for heart disease: the hard-driving, time-conscious, competitive, self-denying, perfectionistic, overachieving "Type A" personality. We were not surprised when our 1985 Survey found that polio survivors reported 50 percent more Type A behavior than did nondisabled individuals. We included the Type A questionnaire in both the 1990 and 1995 International Post-Polio Surveys and had similar results. Of three thousand individuals surveyed, polio survivors reported 30 percent more Type A behavior on average than did individuals of similar age, gender, and income without disabilities. We were relieved when the 1985 Survey found that polio survivors reported no higher rate of heart disease or high blood pressure than did other Americans. However, we also discovered that the more Type A behaviors polio survivors reported, the more new fatigue and muscle pain they were experiencing. And while we had expected to find that physical overexertion and exercise were the most common triggers for fatigue, weakness, and pain, we were unprepared when the Survey uncovered that emotional stress was the *second* most common trigger for PPS symptoms. These findings revealed a disturbing Polio Paradox:

THE WAY OF LIFE ADOPTED BY POLIO SURVIVORS TO HIDE DISABILITY AND BECOME "NORMAL" ACTUALLY TRIGGERS PPS.

It makes sense that polio survivors are more Type A than non-polio survivors. The polio experience provided the ideal environment for becoming Type A. Low self-esteem, loss of control, and lack of social support are all thought to promote Type A behaviors, which are believed to protect against punishment in individuals who are constantly struggling to overcome physical barriers and opposition by others.

To see whether polio survivors had low self-esteem and felt opposed by others, our 1995 Survey included a questionnaire we developed that measures sensitivity to criticism and failure. We found that the polio survivors surveyed were 15 percent more sensitive to the criticism of others and more prone to think of themselves as failures than were the respondents who had not had polio and did not have a disability. Not surprisingly, the more sensitive polio survivors were to criticism and failure, the more Type A behavior they reported. Justice William O. Douglas foretold this finding at least eighty years before our Survey:

I felt ashamed of my appearance, becoming self-conscious and shy, quite irritable and sensitive to all criticism. I came very close to making the perfect scholastic record which I had set as a goal. Yet even this achievement was not enough. For by boyhood standards, I was still crippled, unable to compete physically. By these standards, I was a failure.

Apparently, polio survivors learned and used Type A behavior to prevent criticism by others and to protect against their own feelings of failure.

SUFFERING SERVANTS

We also found that protecting against criticism and failure is more important to polio survivors than is their own emotional or physical well-being. Our 1995 Survey also asked polio survivors if they "Often do what others expect regardless of how you feel emotionally or physically." Nearly three-quarters of those surveyed said yes. And it was no surprise that those answering yes reported 20 percent more Type A behavior and scored more than 50 percent higher in sensitivity to criticism and failure than did survivors who said no. For most polio survivors, it's more important to appear normal and take care of others to protect themselves against criticism and failure than it is to physically and emotionally care for themselves:

> It boils down to either using every ounce of my energy to lead a normal, successful life or giving in to my weaknesses and being inferior. If I fail at anything, I might as well die.
>
> JUDY, CLASS OF '53

> Don't let any polio survivor tell you they just want to "be normal like everyone else." We have to be better than everyone else just to break even . . . and that may not be enough!
>
> MARGARET, CLASS OF '42

Said one of our first patients, Sister Peggy Ryan, O.P.: "Polio survivors aren't just Type A, we're Type E: We do everything for everybody every minute of every day!"

Unfortunately, polio survivors have paid a high price for being Type E, for trying to appear "normal" to escape criticism, failure, and "mortal danger." Type A polio survivors have lived lives of constant vigilance and anxiety, using highly developed "radar" to continuously monitor others' needs and their own performance in an effort to survive, and in the hope of being accepted.

Unfortunately, despite these efforts, polio survivors do not feel accepted. A 1997 study of our patients found that the more Type A polio survivors were, the lonelier they felt and the lower their sense of adequacy, self-worth, and value—as individuals, as family members, and as members of society. Thus another Polio Paradox:

THE TYPE A BEHAVIORS THAT WERE SUPPOSED TO MAKE POLIO SURVIVORS FEEL "NORMAL" AND ACCEPTED ACTUALLY MAKE THEM FEEL MORE LONELY AND UNACCEPTABLE.

So Type A behavior works against polio survivors both physically and emotionally. Survivors' drive to do for others causes them to be so constantly busy that they have no time or energy to be with others. In this way Type A behavior may itself increase loneliness, prevent social support, and thereby promote even *more* Type A behavior.

NOT ALONE IN LONELINESS

Polio survivors are not alone in their responses as adults to the effects of childhood illness, hospitalization, and early-onset disability. German psychiatrist Kathrin Asper has described the lifelong effects of hospitalization in individuals who did not have polio, but who experienced "paralysis, pain and frightening procedures while being cared for by distant and sometimes abusive staff" during long separations from families. Asper discovered that young patients who were not treated with concern by medical staff developed a lifelong aversion to medical treatment and to doctors, as well as an aversion to caring for themselves. These individuals lack compassion for and demand the impossible from themselves. They are out of touch with their own needs but respond to others' needs. Asper thinks they cannot request or accept help because they unknowingly fear repetition of their early experiences of abuse at the hands of people who were supposed to help them. Asper could have been describing the survivors of polio.

So it's not surprising that respondents to our 1995 Survey who *were* treated with concern and whose questions of medical personnel were answered with concern, were almost 10 percent *less* Type A and sensitive to criticism and failure than were polio survivors in general. Nor is it surprising that polio survivors hospitalized later in life for surgeries were nearly 10 percent more Type A and about 5 percent more sensitive to criticism and failure than other polio survivors. It's also understandable that polio survivors who experienced any type of abuse—emotional, physical, or sexual—are about 20 percent more Type A and sensitive to criticism and failure than other polio survivors.

From Kathrin Asper's work, you might think that all adults who experienced early-onset physical disability, were taken from their parents, hospitalized at an early age, and had surgery would be Type A. Yet no other group of people with disabilities has been found to have such a consistent style of behavior as polio survivors. We surveyed adults who had spina bifida, a condition in which children are born with a spinal cord that doesn't "close," leaving many with one or both legs weakened or paralyzed and requiring at least one surgery in infancy. Our survey found that adults with spina bifida were only 1 percent more Type A than individuals without disabilities, while polio survivors were just over 20 percent more Type A than adults with spina bifida.

A "SOCIAL DISEASE"

Apparently, there's something *in addition to* a physical disability early in life, being taken away from parents, being hospitalized, having surgeries—something possibly in addition to the abuse—that caused polio survivors to become so sensitive to criticism and failure and so Type A. I think that this something is polio itself—not polio the disabling disease but polio "The Dread Disease," the AIDS of the middle of the twentieth century:

> I have two personalities: the abused polio child and Superwoman! I would work fourteen-hour days doing my own work and then do other people's work. But I have never felt good enough. I developed this super Type A personality so I wouldn't be abandoned again and rejected like when I had polio.
>
> MARGO, CLASS OF '53

For some polio survivors, no level of activity or accomplishment is sufficient to feel accepted or adequate, let alone valuable:

> I was the best at what I did. Everyone wanted me on their team. I was my boss's favorite and she praised me constantly. But it was never enough. I feel useless and stupid if I'm not doing for others. I get antsy and anxious. I have to work and be seen by everyone to be competent to feel like I'm somebody.
>
> TONI, CLASS OF '48

No level of achievement, no stream of accolades, can make some polio survivors feel that they are anything but unclean and unacceptable, a hobbling child, a paralyzed pariah. This is why I call PPS a social disease—created by polio survivors' response to the expectations, demands, prejudices, and abuses of the society in which they grew up. This is why it's not unusual for our patients never to have discussed their polio experience. Some survivors have never told anyone—not even their spouses or children—that they had polio. Some of our patients have never even spoken the "P word."

When the reality of PPS can no longer be hidden, some polio survivors find themselves more terrified than when they had polio. This is why getting polio survivors to change their Type A ways in order to treat PPS is so difficult.

The Best and the Brightest

Polio survivors heard society's call to normalcy and overshot the mark by a mile. Despite society's negative expectations, nearly three-quarters of polio survivors in our 1985 Survey reported that they were married at the time of the survey, versus about 60 percent of the general population and that they had nearly four years of college on average, versus a high school education for the majority of Americans.

But it's not just American polio survivors who have transcended normalcy. Norwegian researchers have proclaimed polio survivors "well educated and hard working," finding that their years of education, employment, and annual income are the same as workers without disabilities. Anna-Lisa Thoren-Jonsson found that Swedish polio survivors' rate of employment was unrelated to the severity of their disabilities. And polio researcher Frank Lonnberg found that more than 40 percent of polio survivors work overtime and take fewer sick days than nondisabled workers.

But answering the call to normalcy was not limited to American and Scandinavian polio survivors. Patients who come to The Post-Polio Institute for treatment are remarkably similar, whether they are from the Midwest or the Middle East, Belfast or Beijing, South America or South Africa. Normal? Polio survivors from around the globe have transcended mere normalcy to become the world's best and brightest. In addition to an American president, here is just a partial list of the "World's Who's Who" of polio survivors:

Olympic athletes Wilma Rudolph, Tenley Albright,
and Ethelda Blaibtrey...
Authors Arthur C. Clarke and Ben Bradlee...
Actors Mia Farrow, Alan Alda, James Arness,
Donald Sutherland, Christopher Templeton,
and director Francis Ford Coppola...
Dancers Gwen Verdon, Tanaquil Le Clercq,
and Elizabeth Twistington Higgins...
Singers Judy Collins, Joni Mitchell, Neil Young,
Dinah Shore, and Marjorie Lawrence...
Prime Minister Jean Claude Cretien,
Congressmen Fred Grandy and Charles Bennett,
Senator John East, Virginia lieutenant governor John Hager, Sir
Julian Critchley, and Paul Joseph James Martin...
Physicist J. Robert Oppenheimer and physiologist Arthur Guyton...
Founder of M&M Mars chocolate company Frank Mars...
Photographers Lord Snowdon and Dorothea Lange...
U.S. Supreme Court Justice William Orville Douglas...
Violinist Itzhak Perlman...
Golfer Jack Nicklaus...
and you.

Polio survivors discarded polio along with the assistive devices
that allowed them to walk away from the hospital and disappeared into society, telling no one they had been tainted by The
Dread Disease. Polio survivors became Type A overachievers,
successful at everything they did. They became Type E to meet
the needs of everyone—except themselves—and suffered the
constant anxiety of being exquisitely sensitive to criticism and
thinking they had failed.

Of course the ultimate price polio survivors have paid for
becoming "normal" is PPS. As we now turn to the post-polio
body and the cause, treatment, and management of PPS, we
will—we must—return to the post-polio mind, since the late-
onset physical sequelae of polio cannot be treated without
addressing the psychological sequelae of polio and PPS.

PART TWO

"The Beginning of the End?"

CHAPTER 8

Polio Redux?

It's ten minutes of 11 P.M. and I am sitting in a television studio not much bigger than my kitchen. It's 1985 and this is the "big event" that we've been hoping for: For the first time PPS will be introduced to a national television audience.

On the monitor in front of me appears a mop of red hair and a familiar boyish face.

"Dr. Bruno. This is Ted Koppel in Washington. Can you hear me?"

"Yes I can, Ted. It's nice to almost meet you."

Koppel smiles and says, "Dr. Sabin. This is Ted Koppel. Can you hear me?"

In my earpiece booms the voice of Albert Sabin, the developer of the oral polio vaccine: "I don't care if I can hear you. I want to hear Bruno in New York. My hearing isn't what it used to be."

I promise Dr. Sabin I'll speak up. The monitor goes dark and lights again. Over black-and-white newsreel film of children in braces, wheelchairs, and iron lungs, and new color footage of thirty-something polio survivors, I hear, "Why are so many one-time polio victims reporting symptoms that sound like a recurrence of the disease? Good evening. This is Ted Koppel in Washington and this . . . is . . . *Nightline*."

Theme music up. Then it fades and Koppel returns: "This is an alarming echo of what once was, cropping up again . . . what has become a modern medical mystery."

Koppel asks Sabin what he thinks is causing new symptoms.

"I doubt it represents a recurrence of poliovirus activity in the spinal cord," Sabin says. "My impression is that there may be two kinds of post-polio syndrome: one in older people, coming on slowly, who lose more nerve cells with age and, combined with the number of nerve cells that they lost without knowing when they had polio many years ago, you have a combination now that gives rise to weakness or paralysis."

So far so good, I think. Sabin has come to the same conclusion we have, based on his own work and David Bodian's research in the 1940s. New muscle weakness has nothing to do with the poliovirus, but occurs when remaining motor neurons die. But Sabin then goes where no one has gone before:

"The patients that I saw on the screen tonight were young people. It is not likely that they are people who are losing nerve cells now in the spinal cord except, possibly, as a result of infection by biologically related viruses—related to polio—that also can destroy nerve cells."

Oh my God! Fifty-eight seconds into the interview and Albert Sabin has just told America's 1.63 million polio survivors in their forties, fifties, and sixties that they are infected by an unknown virus that's killing their nerves.

I quickly jump in and say that there is no evidence that the poliovirus or *any* other biologically related virus has anything to do with polio survivors' new symptoms. We go on with the discussion as I worry that a dangerous, if nonexistent, cat has been let out of the bag.

Although polio survivors may have been disturbed to hear Albert Sabin opine about an unknown virus causing PPS, such speculation was understandable. A virus caused polio. Why couldn't the poliovirus—even "biologically related viruses"—be responsible for new muscle weakness in polio survivors?

I have to admit that however frightening and unfounded in 1985, a viral cause for PPS makes a great story:

In the 1940s and 1950s an invading virus terrorizes the world year after year. Each wave of invaders kills or disables tens of thousands of people, mainly children. And then the invaders are stopped by a vaccine. The entire world, even those who had been attacked, forgets about the invaders. Those who survive recover and grow up to become, regardless of their disabilities, the country's most prominent and productive citizens . . . even one country's leader.

But wait! But the invaders haven't all gone. Snipers have been left behind. And they wait forty years to begin the attack once more, silently this time, without those who have been invaded even realizing that they are being attacked once again.

Yes, a great story. But is it true? At the same time that PPS symptoms were being reported, new tools were becoming available that would allow researchers to find out. Just over a dozen studies have looked for evidence that the poliovirus can lie dormant in the spinal cord, waiting to begin killing motor neurons once again. In those studies, researchers did spinal taps, collecting the fluid that bathes the spinal cord and the brain, on more than two hundred polio survivors who were reporting new symptoms. Antibodies to the poliovirus or actual pieces of poliovirus were found in the spinal fluid in, at most, 21 percent of polio survivors who had PPS, and in a few polio survivors without new symptoms. The poliovirus pieces were noninfective—they were simply chunks of poliovirus protein and could not infect, reproduce inside of, or kill motor neurons, either in the polio survivors in whom the pieces were found or in anyone else.

Do these antibodies and pieces indicate that the poliovirus does cause new symptoms in polio survivors? No. What Albert Sabin said on *Nightline* was right: PPS is not caused by "a recurrence of poliovirus activity in the spinal cord." If poliovirus were lying in wait to kill off remaining motor neurons, you would

expect many more than 21 percent of polio survivors with PPS—
if not *all* those with new symptoms—to have poliovirus antibodies and protein pieces. Poliovirus antibodies do not indicate
that there is a new infection; they may just be the immune
system's response to the poliovirus pieces.

And the pieces themselves? In 1995 virologist M. E. Leon-
Monzon, who herself found antibodies or poliovirus pieces in
only about 10 percent of those with PPS, concluded that pieces
of poliovirus had been "harbored in some motor neurons that
survived after the acute infection," and that only a small percentage of those with PPS "shed" pieces when the motor neurons
die and break apart.

That's exactly what we thought back in 1985 when the first
study reporting poliovirus antibodies was published. We predicted that pieces of poliovirus protein would also be discovered—what we called the "Take Out the Garbage" Theory. I
wrote that virus pieces would remain inside motor neurons that
had recovered after poliovirus infection—neurons that are now
releasing those pieces as they die, because they can no longer
take the strain of having been damaged, oversprouted, and
turning on double-sized muscle fibers for forty years. The presence of antibodies and poliovirus pieces is thus a secondary
effect of new muscle weakness, not its cause. I'll introduce you
to other findings, including some of our own, that represent
secondary effects of forty-year-old poliovirus damage to neurons.

So whenever you read remarkable reports that explain the
"true cause" of PPS or that propose surefire cures, you have to
take them with a large grain of salt. Many findings are never
confirmed by other researchers. Some findings are statistically
significant—that is, not due to chance—but have absolutely no
meaning in terms of the functioning of your body or the cause
or treatment of PPS. Some studies just aren't done very well,
while other claims are not backed by any research at all. So
please be careful. The truth about PPS is out there; it just isn't
everywhere.

Biologically Related Viruses?

But what about Sabin's second statement, that polio survivors in their fifties are getting weaker because they "are losing nerve cells now in the spinal cord . . . as a result of infection by biologically related viruses—related to polio—that also can destroy nerve cells"? One researcher has found a biologically related virus inside polio survivors' spinal fluid. British virologist Peter Muir has hunted for antibodies and poliovirus pieces in more polio survivors than has anyone else. Although he has concluded that there is no relationship between the poliovirus and PPS, he did detect another member of the enterovirus family—the Coxsackie virus—in the spinal fluid and spinal cords of three polio survivors. What's interesting about Coxsackie viruses is that they can cause damage to the brain and spinal cord that is *identical* to polio. Muir concludes that no virus, neither a dormant poliovirus nor any other, has anything to do with PPS. But the Coxsackie viruses have been suggested as a cause of chronic fatigue syndrome. So here is our first clue that polio, PPS, and CFS may be related—a clue I'll follow up on in chapter 17.

What's in a Name?

Polio survivors' new symptoms are not "polio redux"—not a reawakening of the original poliovirus hiding for decades, nor infection by some other virus. I mentioned in chapter 2 that new symptoms are not a new disease, such as ALS. In fact, new symptoms are not a disease at all. So if they're not "polio redux" and not a new disease we can name, what should we call late-onset symptoms in polio survivors?

Unfortunately, dangers abound when you start naming something you don't fully understand. Thirty years ago neurologist Donald Mulder linked new muscle weakness in polio survivors to muscle atrophy. In the early 1980s, the notion of weakness combining with atrophy gave rise to the moniker post-poliomyelitis progressive muscular atrophy (PPMA or PPPMA).

PPMA implied that polio survivors become weaker as their muscles become smaller. Although a small study by researcher Birgit Abom found that polio survivors' more affected thigh muscles were about half an inch smaller in circumference, very few of our patients have muscles that shrink noticeably over time. When we find atrophy, it's usually in the muscle at the bottom of the thumb. And even documented muscle atrophy is hardly ever associated with muscle weakness. So beware this Post-Polio Fiction:

YOU CAN'T HAVE PPS BECAUSE YOU DON'T HAVE MUSCLE ATROPHY.

Atrophy should be considered a warning sign that neurons are overworking, sprouts are breaking off, or neurons are dying, since muscles get smaller when their motor neurons go away. But you can have new muscle weakness *without* atrophy.

So if *PPMA* doesn't cut it as a name for polio survivors' new symptoms, what would? In 1984, doctors met for the first time at an international symposium to discuss "The Late Effects of Poliomyelitis." But around the same time polio survivors' new symptoms got a catchy new name: *post-polio syndrome*. The name has several different definitions, all based on the notion that only paralytic polio survivors experiencing new muscle weakness can have the "syndrome." But muscle weakness is far from the only symptom polio survivors report. In all of our Post-Polio Surveys, fatigue is the most commonly reported symptom, and survivors of both paralytic and "nonparalytic" polio can have one or any combination of new symptoms: fatigue, muscle weakness, joint and muscle pain, cold intolerance, difficulty sleeping, swallowing, and breathing. So there is no consistent group of symptoms that could be called a "syndrome."

What's more, there are dangers in using *post-polio syndrome* as the name for polio survivors' new problems. Survivors have been told by doctors that there's nothing wrong with them because they didn't have paralytic polio or don't have weakness, and therefore don't meet the definition of "post-polio syndrome." So remember this Post-Polio Precept:

DON'T LET A DOCTOR TELL YOU NOTHING IS WRONG BECAUSE YOU DON'T MEET A DEFINITION OF "POST-POLIO SYNDROME."

Another danger in using *post-polio syndrome* is that it artificially divides polio survivors in research studies into two groups. Nearly all of the research we will be discussing separates polio survivors into those with "post-polio syndrome" and those without. Separating polio survivors using *post-polio syndrome* and its requirement of muscle weakness makes little sense when you're trying to understand new symptoms that have nothing to do with weakness, such as difficulty staying awake during the day, trouble focusing attention, cold intolerance, and difficulty sleeping. This is why our research has studied polio survivors' specific symptoms, and has not divided subjects into "post-polio syndrome" haves and have-nots.

Polio: The Sequel

So if new symptoms are not a syndrome, not PPMA or PPPMA, what *should* they be called? Once again it was David Bodian who asked us to think clearly. Because none of the names adequately describes what is happening to polio survivors, Bodian suggested this: Since all new symptoms came decades after the poliovirus attack, they should be called what they are, the "sequel" to polio—that is, post-polio sequelae. When the International Post-Polio Task Force met in Boston in November 1994, we agreed to use this all-encompassing name. Unfortunately, few people knew what *sequelae* meant, and even fewer could pronounce or spell the word. Doctors and reporters could pronounce *syndrome*, though, and *post-polio syndrome* is the name that stuck. But when you see the initials *PPS* here, I mean *post-polio sequelae*—referring to all of the symptoms polio survivors are now experiencing. And in order to understand all of the symptoms, each needs to be looked at separately. We need to discuss how the poliovirus set the stage for their emergence more than forty years after the poliovirus attack, their triggers, which symptoms can be treated using medication or other therapies, and which must be managed day to day or even hour to hour.

So let's talk about the cause, treatment, and management of PPS. To quote one well-known polio survivor: "We have nothing to fear but fear itself."

CHAPTER 9

The Power Lifter's Lament

They say polio survivors tend to be hard-driving, pressured, time-conscious overachievers. I fit that profile perfectly. After I recovered from the polio I had when I was three, I refused to use a wheelchair or braces, even though my legs were weak. The way I looked was important to me. Physical strength was important, too. So a few years back, I began to power lift. I would spend three days a week doing five-hundred-pound leg presses at the gym thinking I would make my legs stronger and keep them strong. Within two years my legs got weaker. I fell down a flight of stairs and had two surgeries to fix torn ligaments in my feet. Four months later I fell in the shower and broke three toes. I stopped lifting and had to use crutches outside my house. I thought if I could just keep walking I'd get stronger. I didn't know what else to do.

GARY, CLASS OF '48

For polio survivors like Gary, it's déjà vu all over again. For no apparent reason his muscles were becoming weaker. Muscles he had worked so hard to make strong, muscles that had allowed him to be "normal" for decades, were failing him. In our 1985 Survey more than 80 percent of polio survivors reported weakness in muscles paralyzed or weakened during their original bout with polio. Unexpectedly, nearly half reported weakness in muscles that seemed to have been unaffected by polio. And more than 90 percent of polio survivors in the 1985 Survey, as Gary's experience shows, reported that muscle weakness was triggered by physical overexertion and exercise.

Besides unexpected and unexplained muscle weakness, there were additional mysteries. The 1985 Survey found that muscle weakness was triggered by emotional stress in more than 60 percent of polio survivors surveyed and by cold temperatures in more than half. What was going on inside survivors' bodies to cause new muscle weakness?

Death of a Neuron

I have good news and bad news. Let's start with the bad: Polio survivors are getting weaker because their motor neurons are browning out, blacking out, breaking up, and dying. Yes, neurons are dying.

The most sobering and most important study on muscle weakness in polio survivors was performed by Canadian neurophysiologist Alan McComas. McComas actually did two studies using the electromyograph, the EMG, a device measuring the electrical activity that occurs when a motor neuron makes a muscle contract. In the first study McComas used a special EMG technique he himself had developed to count the number of motor neurons remaining after a polio attack. He discovered that muscles known to have been affected by polio had lost 60 percent of their motor neurons, while muscles thought not to have been affected by polio had lost 40 percent. These were exactly the same percentages David Bodian had found fifty years earlier. He discovered that at least 60 percent of motor neurons had to be killed by the poliovirus for a muscle to become weakened, while muscles thought not to have been affected silently lost 40 percent of their motor neurons. McComas confirmed Bodian's finding and this Post-Polio Precept:

THERE IS NO SUCH THING AS AN UNAFFECTED MUSCLE IN SOMEONE WHO HAD PARALYTIC POLIO.

McComas's second study was equally revealing but more disturbing. He counted motor neurons in a group of polio survivors and brought them back for retesting two years later. Over those two years, almost 80 percent reported losing muscle strength. McComas found that they had lost an average of 14 percent of their remaining motor neurons during that time. Being in their midfifties, the polio survivors should not have lost any motor neurons. Most alarming were the findings in the two polio survivors who'd lost the most muscle strength: Each had lost 50 percent of their remaining motor neurons over those two years. McComas found that the more muscle weakness polio survivors experience over time, the more motor neurons are dying.

Why are motor neurons dying? Probably because polio-damaged neurons are severely overworked, having "pumped iron" in one way or another for decades. As we discussed in chapter 3, polio survivors' individual muscle fibers grew, just as they do in weight lifters, and are on average twice the size of fibers in those who've never had polio. These fibers look abnormal—they appear "moth eaten" and show damage typically found only in heavy weight lifters. What's more, the remaining motor neurons turn on about sixteen times more muscle fibers than in someone with no history of polio, thanks to sprouting. Several studies have found that the number of muscle fibers activated by a single post-polio motor neuron increases by about 14 percent each year—twice the percentage of motor neurons McComas found are dying in polio survivors who are becoming weaker. Apparently, as some motor neurons die, their already overworked compatriots sprout to take over the newly orphaned muscle fibers. As polio survivors age, their remaining, damaged, already overworked motor neurons are forced to turn on more and more of the oversized muscle fibers.

Old Neurons: Sprouting and Shrinking

But there are problems besides overwork when middle-aged motor neurons sprout. Older motor neurons are less able to make sprouts—and when they do, the sprouts are thinner and are not covered with myelin, the fatty insulation separating one sprout from another. What's more, fewer muscle fibers are reconnected by the new sprouts, and less of the neurochemical acetylcholine—the chemical that "tells" muscle fibers to contract—is released. And even if the sprouts were insulated, thick and fully functioning, the muscle fibers they are supposed to turn on are not. Everyone who gets older, not just polio survivors, loses muscle fibers. Remaining fibers atrophy, get smaller in size. And aging muscle is not as pliable or as able to contract quickly as is younger muscle. These changes cause a loss of muscle size and strength, reduce muscle contraction speed, and decrease muscle endurance. These effects of aging can further overwork polio survivors' decreasing number of damaged motor neurons and also reduce muscle strength.

Unfortunately, polio survivors' motor neurons are both aging and abnormal, inside and out. A handful of autopsies have been performed in recent years on polio survivors who died more than forty years after having had polio and who reported muscle weakness late in life. Those survivors' remaining, poliovirus-damaged motor neurons were found to be smaller in size and their axons thinner than normal. What's more, the protein factories inside their motor neurons—the same factories that were damaged during the original poliovirus infection—were seen to be breaking apart.

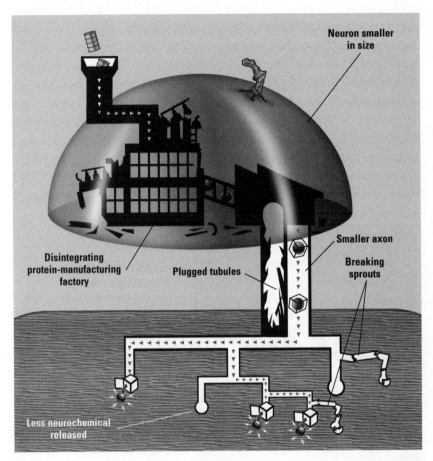

Neuron smaller in size

Smaller axon

Breaking sprouts

Disintegrating protein-manufacturing factory

Plugged tubules

Less neurochemical released

FAILING PPS NEURON

Given that physical overexertion is the most common trigger for muscle weakness in polio survivors, it's instructive that destruction of protein-making machinery also occurs in people who've never had polio but whose neurons have been "exhausted by overwork." How could remaining, poliovirus-damaged motor neurons *not* be overworked and exhausted when they've been turning on sixteen times more double-sized muscle fibers for over forty years?

Yet another problem is seen inside motor neurons of polio survivors who had muscle weakness. A partial plugging of the tubules inside the neuron—the microscopic pipes that carry nutrients and neurochemicals to and from the body of the neuron all the way down to the sprouts—is left over from the original poliovirus infection. So aging, overworked neurons in polio survivors may not only have trouble making mass quantities of protein to support their huge network of sprouts and turn on giant muscle fibers, but also are less able to transport protein quickly throughout the neuron and down to the muscle fibers themselves. Even without plugged pipes, aging neurons in those who never had polio make less protein and move it more slowly.

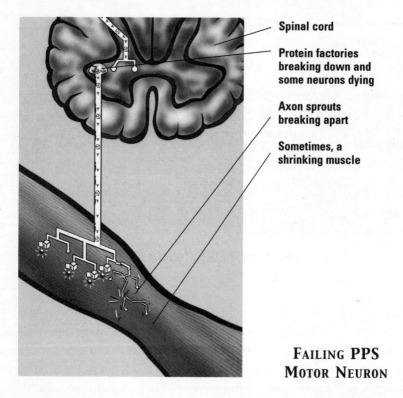

Spinal cord

Protein factories
breaking down and
some neurons dying

Axon sprouts
breaking apart

Sometimes, a
shrinking muscle

**FAILING PPS
MOTOR NEURON**

Alan McComas believes that it is this combination—over-sprouting, overworking, and reduced manufacturing and transportation of protein—that prematurely kills off poliovirus-damaged motor neurons. And he points out that it may not be a coincidence that motor neurons fail and die more frequently in former "iron pumping" athletes like Gary, whether or not they had polio. But Gary isn't the only polio survivor athlete. Given what the poliovirus did to the spinal cord, the amazing extent to which polio survivors' motor neurons compensated for the damage done, and the degree to which survivors have recovered strength and then overused their neurons and muscles, *all* polio survivors should consider themselves athletes!

Breaking Up Isn't Hard to Do

And, yes, there's even more bad news. A small number of polio survivors who report muscle weakness have been tested over the course of several years using a technique called macro EMG, which measures just how much motor neurons sprouted after the polio attack. Polio survivors with progressive weakness have been found to be losing sprouts from year to year. Apparently some polio-damaged neurons are trying to save themselves, like a tree starved for food, by letting branches die off. Because the damaged, overloaded neuron is unable to supply protein to all those extra sprouts, the newest and thinnest "branches" fall off to save the bigger, original branches closest to the "trunk." Is it any wonder that the remaining, damaged motor neurons—over-sprouted and overworked, undernourished and undersized—are breaking up and even dying, and that polio survivors are feeling weaker?

Experience versus Experiments

There is no question that polio survivors' muscles are in fact getting weaker. Ten studies, lasting from nine months to eleven years, have measured muscle strength using either computerized muscle-testing equipment or a manual muscle test, in which doctors or therapists ask you to push or pull against their hands and your strength is rated on a zero-to-five scale. Six studies found that polio survivors who were tested by machine lost on average 5 percent of their muscle strength each year, while those tested by hand lost about 1 percent.

What's more, it's not just strength that polio survivors are losing. Four studies have found that polio survivors' muscles have less endurance (the amount of time a muscle can work before losing strength) and recover strength more slowly after an activity—from hours to days longer than in those who've never had polio. Polio survivors also exert more effort and take longer to perform regular daily activities, such as standing up, walking, and climbing stairs.

THE GOOD NEWS

At this point you may well wonder if there *is* any good news. Well, here it comes. Even polio survivors with only about 50 percent of the neurons they were born with—neurons doing sixteen times more work than before the polio attack and activating muscle fibers twice the size that they should be—don't always become weak. And four studies found *no* muscle weakness in polio survivors who reported that they were losing strength, using either manual or machine muscle testing. Despite all the bad news, there would seem to be a reserve still available in some polio survivors' damaged and severely overloaded motor neurons.

However muscle testing can be deceiving. Any muscle test is only a snapshot in time of a polio survivor's true strength. Even studies using sensitive machines found that any loss of strength is usually very slow, very small, and therefore hard to measure. And studies from the 1950s found that polio survivors who have normal strength when tested by hand are as much as 55 percent weaker when tested by machine. So a normal manual muscle test in your doctor's office doesn't mean you have normal strength.

So it's not unusual that patients who return to The Post-Polio

Institute reporting that they feel weaker, have poorer balance, are walking less far and less well—are even falling down—are found to have strength on a manual muscle test that has not changed from the year before. So beware this Post-Polio Fiction:

IF A MANUAL MUSCLE TEST SHOWS NORMAL STRENGTH, YOU SHOULDN'T BE FEELING WEAKER AND CAN'T HAVE PPS.

Regardless of its results, no manual muscle test measures your endurance, effort, or the time it takes for you to recover strength after activity. And as polio survivors know well, muscle weakness—indeed, *all* PPS symptoms—changes from day to day and sometimes from hour to hour. Transient muscle weakness, those up-and-down changes in strength, won't necessarily be picked up in your doctor's office even during monthly visits. All in all, your own experience of muscle weakness, endurance, effort, and ability to function are the best measures of whether you're losing strength.

THE POST-POLIO ROLLER COASTER

Unfortunately, the lack of attention to transient weakness in polio survivors is a shortcoming of all the muscle strength studies I've mentioned. Many researchers and treating doctors have approached PPS as if it were a disease. We said PPS is not a disease. If it were, all the studies would have consistently found measurable and progressive muscle weakness in polio survivors, as is seen in ALS. Muscle weakness in polio survivors is in fact more subtle and much more variable. Even more unfortunate is that polio survivors themselves don't pay attention to transient weakness:

If the accepted theory of post-polio muscle weakness is that motor neurons are dying, why do I improve with rest after having a period of severe weakness after I overdo? Even though I can become completely lame for a day, the weakness is temporary if I rest up. My doctor tested my muscles and I am no weaker this year than last. I can't be doing any harm if the doctor finds my muscles are strong when he tests them.

FIONA, CLASS OF '47

Like too many polio survivors, Fiona thinks it's okay to ride the post-polio roller coaster: Work until you crash, rest long enough to be able to function, and then work again until you crash. As Gary found out, you can't keep exhausting your neurons over and over without paying a stiff price. A loss of strength after you've done too much—especially if you're not able to use a muscle at *all*—is a clear warning sign that something dangerous is happening inside your motor neurons. Even transient weakness means that your neurons have been overloaded and drained of their protein and nutrient reserves. Think of what would happen to your car's battery if you left the headlights on every night. You'd wake up the first morning with a flat battery. You'd get a jump start and drive off. You leave the lights on again the second night, wake to a flat battery, get a jump start again the next day, and drive away. After about a week, though, the battery would no longer take a charge, and you wouldn't be driving anywhere! You can replace your car's dead battery, but you can't replace your motor neurons. Even though rest allows Fiona's neurons to recover and muscle strength returns, Alan McComas's research and our own clinical experience at The Post-Polio Institute says that every time polio survivors exhaust their motor neurons, they are doing damage that will eventually result in permanent weakness. Neurons will no longer recover from exhaustion, their sprouts may break off, and they simply die. We have several patients who have literally pushed their motor neurons over the edge. They did too much for too long, ignored transient and even progressive loss of strength, and now have permanent and disabling muscle weakness.

EXPERIMENTING VERSUS TREATING

I have some more good news. A very important problem with the experiments measuring polio survivors' muscle strength is that not one of them compared polio survivors who were being treated for new muscle weakness to those who weren't. So the studies don't tell us if polio survivors would still lose muscle strength if they were doing something to take the load off their neurons.

However, one study is different. Physiatrist Paul Peach asked patients he had treated for PPS to return for a reevaluation. He conducted manual muscle tests and found that his patients had lost 1.5 percent of their muscle strength over two years, about the same amount of loss that had been found in other studies. But Peach knew that not all polio survivors were alike in their willingness to accept the treatments he recommended to take the load off poliovirus-damaged neurons. So he split his patients into three groups: those who did not comply with any of his PPS treatment recommendations, those who partially complied, and those who fully complied. Polio survivors who didn't comply with any recommendations lost 4 percent of their muscle strength over the next two years; those who partially complied lost about 3 percent, while those who fully complied actually gained just over 1 percent per year. This study contains the best news and the most hopeful Post-Polio Precept of all:

THE ONLY CAUSE OF PROGRESSIVE MUSCLE WEAKNESS IS POLIO SURVIVORS NOT TAKING CARE OF THEMSELVES.

Peach's findings dovetail with the results of our 1997 study, in which we sent anonymous surveys asking about symptoms to all of the post-polio patients we had treated to date. Polio survivors who refused to begin or who left treatment reported 60 percent more muscle weakness sixteen months later. At this point in The Post-Polio Institute's ongoing Treatment Outcome Study, just one month after completing our treatment program, partially compliant patients report 10 percent more muscle weakness, while fully compliant patients report 11 percent *less* weakness. When it comes to stopping the progression of muscle weakness, your neurons are in your own hands.

Diagnosis of Exclusion

Just what are the treatment recommendations that actually help polio survivors gain strength? Before we talk about treating muscle weakness, we have to make sure that weakness is in fact a PPS symptom. Hence this essential Post-Polio Precept:

ALL PPS ARE DIAGNOSED BY *EXCLUSION*.

"Diagnosed by exclusion" means that your doctor has to perform tests to exclude all other possible causes for muscle weakness—and for all symptoms that you think might be PPS—before concluding by a process of elimination that your symptoms are PPS. A process of exclusion is needed because, despite more than twenty years of research, there is still not *one* test that can prove new muscle weakness or any other new symptom is PPS. It had been hoped that the EMG would be *the* tool for diagnosing PPS. And there have been dozens of studies using the EMG to test polio survivors with and without new muscle weakness. However, not one has found that the regular EMG doctors can do in their offices proves you have PPS. So watch out for another Post-Polio Fiction:

YOU CAN'T HAVE PPS BECAUSE YOUR EMG DOESN'T PROVE IT.

The studies showing that motor neurons are dying and breaking up use special EMG techniques performed at university medical centers. Your local doctor doesn't do these special EMGs. What's more, the special EMG studies showing the death and disintegration of motor neurons were conducted over the course of years. Even if you went today to a medical center where a special EMG could be done, you wouldn't know for a year whether your neurons were shrinking or dying.

However, your doctor may want a regular EMG to exclude another cause for your muscle weakness, such as a severely herniated disc pressing on the spinal cord or a nerve, or a neurological disease like ALS. EMGs are both expensive and painful. So before you agree to have one, ask what the doctor is looking for, and make sure that he or she isn't doing an EMG to "prove" you have PPS. What's more, you shouldn't be denied long-term disability or Social Security disability because an EMG didn't prove you have PPS.

If you do have new weakness, is there a chance that you have something other than PPS? Yes, but the chance is very small. In twenty years we've never seen a polio survivor with ALS, nor any with a herniated disc or a rare muscle disease that caused weakness. We have seen six patients who had PPS plus another neurological disease (Parkinson's or Alzheimer's disease), but the other diagnosis was obvious as soon as the patient walked through the door. Again, you must be fully evaluated to exclude all other conditions, neurological and medical, before the diagnosis of PPS is accepted. But there's an old medical adage: "If you hear hoofbeats, expect horses, not zebras." The good news is, if you have new muscle weakness, expect PPS.

POLIO OR NO?

We are sometimes asked if there is a test that proves whether someone had polio at all. For those who aren't sure that they had polio and who never received the polio vaccine, measuring antibodies to the polioviruses might show an increase that would reflect the type of poliovirus that infected you. It's also possible to have a biopsy in which a small piece of muscle is removed to look for evidence of the death and oversprouting of motor neurons. Another source of indirect evidence would be the special EMGs I mentioned; these could show if you'd lost motor neurons or if your remaining motor neurons are oversprouted, suggesting that something had damaged your spinal cord, that "something" most likely being the poliovirus.

The most readily available test that can show if motor neurons have been killed is a regular EMG. But just as a regular EMG can't identify which muscles have new weakness, this test also isn't always able to identify muscles whose motor neurons were damaged during the poliovirus attack. Physiatrist Mark Bromberg found that almost 10 percent of patients who had a history of polio and had muscle weakness, and who were reporting new pain, fatigue, or weakness in midlife, had normal regular EMGs, meaning that there was no EMG evidence they'd ever had polio.

It has been suggested that every polio survivor get a regular EMG to identify muscles that were *not* affected by the poliovirus and to identify which muscles can be exercised without fear that they'll become weaker. One study using regular EMGs found that almost a quarter of paralytic polio survivors' limbs had no evidence of motor neurons having been killed. Those limbs were classified as having "no clinical polio" and could therefore be exercised like anyone else's muscles. However, neurologist Carlos Luciano, using macro EMG, found oversprouted motor neurons in 85 percent of muscles that were thought to have had "no clinical polio." And you already know that research by David Bodian and Alan McComas showed that seemingly unaffected muscles had lost 40 percent of their motor neurons.

The danger of using a regular EMG to diagnose polio or identify "unaffected" muscles comes through loud and clear in the experience of one of our patients, whose legs had been severely weakened by polio and were getting weaker, causing him to walk with crutches. He believed that polio had not affected his arms and he wanted to go on a "walking tour" of Europe. He asked for a regular EMG of all the muscles of his arms, which showed absolutely no evidence of polio. Off he went on his crutches to Europe, where his arms started to become weak; he returned a month later barely able to lift them. The moral is that an expensive and painful EMG is neither reliable nor desirable if you're trying to decide how you should take care of your muscles. The safest thing to do is to assume that every muscle was affected by polio and follow the Post-Polio Precept we call "The Golden Rule"—the fundamental tenet that underlies all PPS treatment:

IF ANYTHING CAUSES FATIGUE, WEAKNESS, OR PAIN, *DON'T DO IT!* (OR DO MUCH LESS OF IT.)

"Nonparalytic" Polio

Many polio survivors have been told this Post-Polio Fiction:

YOU CAN'T HAVE PPS UNLESS YOU HAD PARALYTIC POLIO.

This leaves those with so-called "nonparalytic" polio—those who didn't have weakness or paralysis after the poliovirus attack—out in the cold. Distinguishing between paralytic and "nonparalytic" polio doesn't make sense when you look at what the poliovirus did to the spinal cord and brain. Both David Bodian and Alan McComas have shown us that whether poliovirus damage to motor neurons causes no symptoms, mild weakness, or full-blown paralysis is just a matter of degree. The poliovirus could have killed up to 60 percent of your neurons without your having any muscle weakness, and you could have been diagnosed with "nonparalytic" polio. However, over the years, as polio-damaged neurons fail, "nonparalytic" polio survivors can be pushed over the 60 percent threshold and begin having new muscle weakness.

In 1994 researcher Linda Nee proved the point. She tracked down the North Carolina twins whom C. N. Herndon had studied. One twin in each case had paralytic polio, as you'll recall, and the other had "nonparalytic" polio. Nee found that 70 percent of the twins who had paralytic polio have PPS today. The surprise was that more than 40 percent of the twins who had "nonparalytic" polio—who had no weakness or paralysis at all after the polio attack—also have PPS.

Unfortunately, most polio survivors don't have medical records (as the twins did) to document a diagnosis of "nonparalytic" polio. Some polio survivors never saw a doctor, especially those who lived outside cities and who couldn't easily get to a hospital. More than twice as many cases of "nonparalytic" polio and 15 percent more paralytic cases were reported in people living in cities than among those living in outlying areas.

But even if polio survivors did see a doctor, their diagnoses were not necessarily correct. As early as 1941, David Bodian cautioned that the "diagnosis of a non-paralytic case may rest on the failure to detect minimal degrees of muscle weakness." Thus Bodian predicted the findings of doctors more than a dozen years later on two different coasts. In 1954 New York polio specialists Shaw and Levin found that mild weakness could be easily overlooked if strength was tested only at the bedside: "Many patients who are eager for activity, who can readily walk out of the hospital, and who are persuasively non-paralytic will . . . have very definite muscle weakness which cannot be detected while they are recumbent in bed."

Even those whose strength was evaluated when they were walking may have been misdiagnosed as having "nonparalytic" polio if the evaluation took place within a month or so after their acute polio. California polio specialists Moskowitz and Kaplan found that almost 40 percent of polio survivors who were reexamined up to six years after having been diagnosed with "nonparalytic" polio had weakness in at least one muscle. So even if you were diagnosed with "nonparalytic" polio, or only had weakness in just a few muscles, you can have weakness today in any muscle.

THE BIGGER THEY ARE

There's one last point about which muscles develop weakness. Researcher Jeffery Klingman found that it's the combination of how weak muscles were after the poliovirus attack plus how much strength was recovered that predicts which muscles become weak, not just how weak muscles were to begin with. This makes perfect sense. A muscle that has been weak since 1952 and doesn't do much today doesn't have much strength to lose. But a muscle that was paralyzed and fully recovered, thanks to damaged neurons sprouting and muscle fibers becoming bigger, has been overworking its motor neurons and is more likely to fail. The better and bigger your muscles got, the harder your neurons are going to "fall."

Stress and PPS

Given what we've discussed about having too few polio-damaged, oversprouted, and overworked neurons, it makes sense that physical overexertion and exercise are the most commonly reported triggers for muscle weakness. But why did two-thirds of polio survivors in our 1985 Survey report that muscle weakness was triggered by cold temperatures, and almost half say that muscle weakness was triggered by emotional stress? I'll devote all of chapter 13 to the effects of cold. But let's start to talk about stress right here.

THE STRESS OF TRAUMA

Among polio survivors, three traumatic events combine to produce both physical and emotional stress: illness, injury, and surgery. In 1996 we reviewed the histories of all the polio survivors we had evaluated to date and found that almost 20 percent said their PPS began after a traumatic event. The traumas that triggered new symptoms included pregnancy, illnesses such as pneumonia, chemotherapy, breaking an ankle, leg, or hip, and surgeries, including hip and knee replacements. Polio survivors also experienced falls and auto accidents in which the most common injury—in nearly three-quarters—was to the leg. And one-quarter had had back injuries. Regardless of the type of trauma or its location, the most common symptom was new muscle weakness, reported by just over half of our patients. One-third reported pain, and only about 10 percent reported fatigue.

It was clear that trauma didn't "turn on" PPS, as if it were lying in wait for an opportunity to spring forth. Symptoms also didn't begin in an injured area and then spread throughout the body. Seventy percent of patients had new symptoms only in the area that had been injured, while a quarter had symptoms in the injured area plus one other nearby location. For example, 40 percent of those who injured one leg developed weakness or pain only in the other leg. This is a common situation in polio survivors, who compensate for injury on one side of the body by overusing the same part on the other side. Only 5 percent of patients developed symptoms in more than two areas of their bodies.

And another piece of good news: Regardless of the type of trauma or severity of their injuries, nearly 90 percent of patients had significant reductions in muscle weakness, pain, and fatigue after receiving the same treatment we give to any polio survivor with PPS symptoms. The remaining patients experienced a reduction in some symptoms, especially pain, but continued to report muscle weakness or fatigue. Our patients proved that polio survivors are resilient and will not disintegrate even if they break bones or have surgery. This conclusion is reinforced by the finding that, for each patient who reported new symptoms after trauma, at least one other patient had had the same trauma but did *not* develop new symptoms. So although trauma can be sufficient to cause new symptoms, PPS do not necessarily "cometh after a fall."

EMOTIONAL STRESS

Even without physical injury, illness, or surgery, our 1985 Survey found that emotional stress alone is the second leading trigger of PPS symptoms. Our experience over the years has made clear

that emotional stress is a force to be reckoned with, given its profound ability to trigger fatigue, weakness, and pain:

> I had a minor case of polio with weakness in one leg that
> disappeared. I had always been very active and athletic.
> Then in late 1998 I began experiencing back and leg pain
> as well as general fatigue. Shortly thereafter both my legs
> became quite weak and I had a great deal of difficulty
> walking. I felt emotionally burned out from the over-
> whelming stress of my work, my divorce, and the death of
> my father. I started falling down and generally felt like my
> entire body had fallen into an abyss.
>
> JOHN, CLASS OF '54

> It was a Monday morning and I'd had a very relaxed
> weekend. I went into the weekly meeting feeling rested
> and wide awake. The meeting turned contentious, with
> angry accusations being hurled back and forth and blame
> passed around and around. After three hours the meeting
> broke up. I went to stand and my legs wouldn't hold me! I
> fell back into the chair. They had to bring me lunch and it
> took an hour before I could walk back to my office.
>
> ALLY, CLASS OF '51

Although we don't know exactly how emotional stress triggers
muscle weakness, pain, or fatigue in polio survivors, cortisol may
be the missing link. Cortisol is the body's main antistress hormone. Cortisol is produced by the adrenal glands when you are
under stress, and puts a brake on your neurons so that they don't
get carried away with themselves and allow your blood pressure
and heart rate to go through the roof, leading to a stroke or heart
attack.

But as important as cortisol is to your survival, it's also
harmful. The animal version of cortisol has been shown to slow
or stop the sprouting of motor neurons in studies of aged animals. Studies have also shown that when animals having dam-

aged nerves are stressed, their muscles' endurance is reduced, and there is a decrease in the number of motor neuron sprouts. These effects may be due to cortisol interfering with motor neurons' ability to make proteins and use blood sugar.

Both the symptoms and damaging effects of emotional stress on neurons are excellent reasons for polio survivors to stop stressing—physically and emotionally—their poliovirus-damaged, overworked, and oversprouted motor neurons.

Just Say No to Drugs

Speaking of chemicals, the first question new patients often ask is if there is a drug, some "magic pill," they can take to get stronger and make PPS go away. Alas, no. There have been double-blind, placebo-controlled studies of several drugs to treat muscle weakness: insulinlike growth factor (which is similar to growth hormone), Mestinon, amantadine, and prednisone, a powerful steroid similar to cortisol. Not one medication has been found to increase strength or functional ability in polio survivors. And despite what you may read on the Internet, no studies have shown that herbal remedies or electrical stimulation increase muscle strength. Polio survivors mustn't think that they can run themselves ragged, pop a pill, or plug themselves into some electrical device and make their PPS disappear.

A Weakness for Exercise

After polio survivors ask me if there's a pill to cure muscle weakness, their second request is for exercises to strengthen muscles. And why wouldn't they ask? Weak muscles should be exercised! That's what polio survivors were told when they were recovering from polio, and it's what many doctors tell them today. But does this sound familiar?

My legs had been getting weaker so I joined a gym last summer. After about a month my arms started to get weaker and my back hurt so I stopped going. In January I shoveled snow and my left leg became exhausted. I had trouble walking up the steps into my house. My knee buckled twice but I caught myself before I fell. I went to my doctor and he sent me to physical therapy. In the first session I was on the treadmill for five minutes, on the bike for ten, and I did leg raises with weights around my ankles. I barely made it home, where I fell to the kitchen floor. My legs are even weaker, and now they are twitching and burning.

ROBERTA, CLASS OF '50

Given Gary's and Roberta's experiences, exercise doesn't sound like the cure for post-polio muscle weakness. But treatment for PPS should not be based on patient reports alone, no matter how compelling. The effects of exercise need to be studied. And there have been about half a dozen small studies that on average tested twelve polio survivors' ability to increase strength with exercise. The studies all tested survivors' ability to strengthen the quadriceps muscle, the muscle in the front of your upper leg that lifts your lower leg up off the floor and keeps your leg straight, an activity called knee extension. Knee extension allows you to stand up from a chair and "locks" your knee to prevent you from falling once you're standing. And although 90 percent of the subjects were diagnosed as having "post-polio syndrome" or reported new muscle weakness, their legs were quite strong. While seated, subjects were able to straighten their leg many times with a weight on their ankles.

The strengthening studies differed in length from six weeks to two years, asked polio survivors to exercise from two to four times each week, and were different in the exercises that were prescribed. Most asked polio survivors to lift their leg upward with a weight attached to the ankle or to push against a computerized strength-measuring machine. Two studies limited exercise if polio survivors felt fatigue, asked them to rest between periods of exercise, and increased the amount of weight lifted only if polio survivors reported no "excessive fatigue." Other studies described their exercise regime as "high-intensity," "heavy resistance," or "aggressive." Two studies required that polio survivors spend five minutes warming up on an exercise bicycle before they did as many as thirty leg lifts three times each week. In the most aggressive study, polio survivors did the five minutes of bicycle warm-up, followed by a sixty-minute exercise class twice a week for five months! I have to tell you that a polio survivor who is able, twice a week for five months, to ride five minutes on an exercise bicycle and then complete a sixty-minute exercise class is not someone whose ability to function is being compromised by PPS. The subjects in the studies had more strength, more endurance, more ability to function, and fewer symptoms than our least affected post-polio patients.

Still, when you read the researchers' conclusions, it sounds like exercise is just the thing to restore muscle strength in any polio survivor who has PPS:

> These results demonstrate that a supervised training program can lead to significant gains in strength . . . without muscular damage.

> The training program could be performed without major complications and resulted in an increase in muscle strength.

> After training, a significant increase in strength was observed and maintained for some time.

However, when you look at the responses of individual subjects, the benefits of exercise are far from clear. Just over half of those who exercised had an increase in upper leg muscle strength of about 25 percent. One-quarter had no change in strength, while 20 percent actually had a decrease in strength of about 10 percent. So almost as often as not, exercise either had no effect or actually *decreased* muscle strength.

But there's more—well, actually less. Only two studies asked whether exercise had an impact on polio survivors' ability to function in their daily lives. In a 1996 "low-intensity" muscle strengthening study by physiatrist Jim Agre, where exercise was increased only if subjects felt no increase in exertion, there was no measurable change in muscle strength or endurance, although half the subjects believed that their walking and stair climbing improved. In a more aggressive study in which physiatrist Gisli Einarsson had polio survivors bicycle and then do two dozen leg lifts three times a week for six weeks, there was no increase in the subjects' ability to perform daily activities despite a measured increase in muscle strength of nearly 30 percent. Unfortunately, polio survivors' muscle endurance decreased during the year after the experiment by 300 percent!

I use "the milkmaid" analogy to explain the best-case scenario results of these studies: If polio survivors who are able to lift a gallon of milk five times participate in a muscle-strengthening program, half will become able to lift five quarts of milk, but they will only be able to lift them three times.

This illustrates a Post-Polio Precept:

POLIO SURVIVORS CAN DO ALMOST ANYTHING ONCE.

Many of our patients report that it isn't so much a loss of strength that limits their ability to function but rather a loss of endurance, the ability to keep doing a task, like repetitive lifting and especially walking distance. And while the ability to perform tasks requiring a burst of strength can increase with exercise in some polio survivors, their ability to do things that require endurance, in Gisli Einarsson's words, "fades away."

You have to ask what good comes from an exercise program that produces small increases in muscle strength that are not associated with an increased ability to do daily activities, and that can cause muscle endurance to decrease more than strength increases.

CAN EXERCISE BE HELPFUL?

When should you exercise to strengthen weakened muscles? Never. Alan McComas concluded that "polio survivors should not engage in fatiguing exercise or activities that further stress metabolically damaged neurons that are already overworking."

However, carefully prescribed and monitored *nonfatiguing* exercise may be helpful in a few special situations. If we recommend a short leg brace for patients who can still move their feet, we will sometimes suggest doing nonfatiguing "ankle pumps," in which the foot is moved up and down several times, the idea being not to increase strength but to prevent the weakness that can be caused by a leg being immobilized in a brace for most of the day. What's the definition of *nonfatiguing*? We use the formula described by Canadian physiatrist Rubin Feldman: with the physical therapist watching, a patient does *half* the amount of exercise that causes any symptom, including muscle weakness, fatigue, or pain. Polio survivors are amazed when this piddling amount of exercise maintains the size and strength of their muscle and when muscle strength and endurance actually increase after they begin to use braces. But we never recommend even nonfatiguing exercise for muscles with less than antigravity strength—(those graded "poor" or less than "three") that can't lift their own weight against gravity.

A small percentage of our patients have worn out their joints after years of overuse-abuse, and have had hip and knee replacements. And unfortunately, polio survivors do fall and break bones. After surgery or after a limb comes out of a cast, muscles will be weaker. Carefully monitored, slowly increasing, nonfatiguing exercise can help polio survivors to regain muscle strength. Nonfatiguing exercise is also prescribed when our patients develop "Post-Polio Shoulder"—painful bursitis and tendinitis caused by overuse. Gentle, nonfatiguing exercise to strengthen shoulder muscles is begun, but only after shoulder pain has been treated using ultrasound, heat, massage, and nonsteroidal anti-inflammatory drugs—and, of course, after the patient has stopped the activities causing overuse.

THE CARDIAC CONUNDRUM

One understandable concern of middle-aged polio survivors is heart disease. When polio survivors have clogged arteries or have had a heart attack, cardiologists often tell them to "get out and walk!" But walking, especially at the pace necessary to help the heart stay fit, can exact a hefty price:

> After my heart attack the doctor sent me to cardiac rehabilitation. They put me on "the circuit": five minutes on the bicycle, five on the treadmill, and five on the leg-lift machine. The therapists were mad because I couldn't increase my time on the machines. But my right leg was getting weaker and it was harder and harder to walk. After three months I had to use a cane. I told my cardiologist but he said I had to keep going. Now I can't do one minute on the machines and I have to use two canes because I can hardly use my one leg at all.
>
> LEO, CLASS OF '38

What do you do when you have one body with two conflicting needs: One indispensable muscle needs exercise while all the other muscles need rest? There have been only four studies of heart exercise for polio survivors. One was the very aggressive exercise study mentioned above—where polio survivors did the five minutes of bicycle warm-up followed by a sixty-minute exercise class twice a week for five months. This study found that polio survivors' legs became about 5 percent weaker, their ability to function in their daily lives did not improve, but their highest heart rate during exercise (a measure of how much of a workout the heart is getting) increased by twelve beats per minute. This is another example of the trade-off our patient describes above:

The heart muscle gets a workout while the leg muscles get weaker.

Two other studies of heart exercise were not aggressive at all. The amount of exercise was reduced if polio survivors reported discomfort, pain, or fatigue. Polio survivors pedaled a stationary exercise bicycle with either legs or their arms, but *paced* their exercise, pedaling in intervals of two minutes separated by one-minute rests. In this way, and with fatigue and pain as their guides, polio survivors cycled three times a week for sixteen weeks and were able to increase their pedaling time by the end of the study. Heart rate during exercise increased among those on the leg bicycle by five beats per minute and by eleven beats per minute with the arm bicycle. Arm muscles are smaller than leg muscles, so arm exercise is more taxing on the heart and a more efficient form of heart exercise. Since most polio survivors' legs are weaker than their arms, it's more likely that paced, non-fatiguing arm exercise would be both more effective and more doable by polio survivors who need heart exercise. At The Post-Polio Institute, if patients' fatigue, weakness, and pain remain significantly reduced one month after graduation from the program, we will develop a paced, nonfatiguing arm bicycle exercise program for those with heart disease.

By the same token, polio survivors with muscle weakness or fatigue should not have a cardiac stress test that requires them to walk on a treadmill or ride a bike. Medication can be given, such as the drug adenosine, that shows how open heart muscle arteries are without stressing polio survivors' leg muscles.

IS SWIMMING ALL WET?

Polio survivors often believe that water exercise, which they were given when they had polio, is not only helpful to treat new muscle weakness but also is totally harmless, since the buoyancy of the water reduces gravity and makes it easier to move in the pool. Some polio survivors think that water aerobics, which use the resistance of the water to stress muscles and increase heart rate, is safe because it's done in a pool. But a study by Carin Willen of nonfatiguing water exercise found no increase in heart rate among polio survivors, but did find that their leg strength decreased by nearly 10 percent.

If you are going to get into a pool, it must be warm—more than 85 degrees Fahrenheit or 30 degrees Celsius. Second, you should take advantage of buoyancy and warmth to do stretching, but don't fight against the water's resistance to do walking or fatiguing aerobics. You may be able to use your arms to swim to exercise your heart, but the exercise must be prescribed by your cardiologist and monitored by a rehabilitation doctor and physical therapist knowledgeable about PPS. As with any activity, on land or in the water, The Golden Rule always applies.

LAZY BONES?

Polio survivors are told that two other conditions should be treated with walking: deconditioning and osteoporosis. Many doctors and some polio survivors believe that new weakness and fatigue result from deconditioning, in which the muscles and nerves get "lazy" and stop working because polio survivors lie around too much. Other survivors believe that their currently strong leg muscles will deteriorate unless they walk to prevent deconditioning.

Deconditioning is one of the red herrings that doctors who know nothing about PPS try to feed you. Deconditioning can occur when someone is confined to bed for a week. But in twenty years we have seen only two polio survivors who were deconditioned, both of whom had severe depression.

An exercise program is not required to prevent your muscles from turning to jelly. When my patients worry that they will no longer be able to walk unless they start jogging or join a gym, I ask them to go to a department store and look around. How many of the Golden Agers elbowing you away from the sale items at Wal-Mart do you think run marathons to stay fit? Even polio researcher Jim Agre, a proponent of muscle-strengthening exercise for polio survivors, warns, "For some persons, the performance of normal activities of daily living may require maximal effort, and additional exercise may lead to overuse problems." One of our patients said she feels like she's "run a marathon" every morning just by getting out of bed, washing, and dressing. Yet she believed that she had to keep on keeping on, continue "running the marathon" to prevent herself from getting weaker. An important Post-Polio Precept applies here:

ACTIVITY IS NOT AN EXERCISE PROGRAM.

Ask yourself if you feel stronger on the days you've walked two miles in the mall or stayed home and read the Sunday paper. Just doing more activity—walking farther, climbing more stairs—in the hope that you will become stronger is not an exercise program. It is abuse.

With regard to osteoporosis, since the majority of women we see at The Post-Polio Institute are of menopausal age, losing bone density is bound to be a problem. Although one Mayo Clinic study found that polio survivors have no more osteoporosis than anyone else, this finding makes little sense when you look at polio survivors in general. Bones that bear weight with walking and muscles pulling on bones increases the amount of calcium deposited inside. Polio survivors who had paralysis often have shorter legs, either because they didn't "push" on their legs—didn't stand on them—because they used a weight-bearing brace, crutches, or a wheelchair—or because their weaker muscles didn't "pull" on bones enough to help calcium deposit and allow bones to grow. The same lack of pushing and pulling over the years causes osteoporosis in both women *and* men who have paralysis or just have muscle weakness. Post-polio researcher Margaret Campbell found that women polio survivors lose bone density at a faster rate than women without disabilities. And a Danish study concluded that polio survivors have as much as 50 percent less bone density in their more affected leg.

But taking up walking or other exercise to push and pull on bones is certainly not a treatment for polio survivors' osteoporosis, since walking is a cause of PPS muscle weakness. All menopausal women should have a bone density study—as should men who have paralysis or muscle weakness, use wheelchairs or crutches, or wear braces—to see if they have osteoporosis. Women can talk to their doctors about using hormone replacement to treat bone loss. Both women and men can discuss with their doctors taking calcium supplements and using anti-bone-loss medications, such as Fosamax and calcitonin. We have patients who use wheelchairs and have never walked whose osteoporosis has been significantly decreased through medication alone.

What Then Can You Do?

By now you must be champing at the bit! If there's no magic pill, no miraculous machine, no muscle-strengthening exercise to "cure" muscle weakness, what can polio survivors do to make their muscles stronger and keep them strong?

Unfortunately, you can't manage any PPS symptom in isolation. This is especially true for muscle weakness—which all by itself can cause pain and fatigue—as well as sleeping, swallowing, and breathing problems. We have to look at the whole picture—the whole person and all symptoms—and then map out a head-to-toe plan to treat and manage PPS. Let's press on by discussing PPS that are a pain in the neck . . . and elsewhere.

CHAPTER 10

Pain and the Post-Polio Brain

I don't remember the feeling of paralysis but I do remember the pain. The headache lasted for ten days, which seemed like an eternity to a six-year-old. It throbbed from my eyebrows back over the top of my head and down the back of my neck. Nothing made it better. Sometimes I think I can still feel that headache.

Headaches began again in 1985. I had two or three a week. These headaches were similar to and different from the one during my acute polio. The new headache also went across my head and down the back of my neck. But the new pain reached to my shoulder blades, could be on the left or right side of my head, and made me sick to my stomach. The pain was so severe I could not work. But headaches aren't my only new pain. My first PPS symptom was a constant muscle spasm in my "good" leg. I have also had tendinitis in my right elbow and wrist, and bursitis in my left hip and right shoulder. Sometimes I think I'm a medley of pains!

DEE, CLASS OF '49

Pain was often the first harbinger of polio. The poliovirus caused pain that could engulf the entire body: pounding headaches, burning in the spine, and viselike muscle spasms.

For many polio survivors, the memory of that pain was lost until PPS appeared. In the early 1980s, when polio survivors were first reporting new symptoms, some said they were experiencing pain that was "just like the pain I had with polio." This new pain was frequently associated with aching all over the body. Some doctors thought this whole-body pain was unique to polio survivors, suggested that it was a symptom of a recurrence of the original disease, and dubbed it "post-polio pain."

The notion that there is a unique, whole-body post-polio pain was discarded quickly. Combining patient reports with the results of our Surveys, it became apparent that polio survivors' "whole-body" pain was the result of pain in many separate locations. Our Surveys found that headaches are reported by a third of polio survivors while neck, back, arm, and leg muscle pain occur in nearly three-quarters. Polio survivors report specific triggers for their pain, the most common being physical overactivity and exercise, followed by cold exposure, emotional stress, anxiety, and Type A behavior. But how do these triggers cause pain?

When Good Muscles Go Bad

Headaches, neck pain, and back pain are almost always caused by muscle spasms. To understand muscle spasms, you have to remember what muscles are supposed to do: They contract, becoming shorter, to make your body parts move. Normally your brain tells your muscles to contract to move your legs, or arms, or head, and then tells the muscles to relax so that you stop moving. But there are conditions in which muscles don't turn off after they contract. This sets the stage for painful continuous muscle contractions and then a muscle spasm—the constant, painful shortening and rock-hard "knotting up" of a muscle.

MUSCLE IMBALANCES AND "BRACING"

Many polio survivors have muscle imbalances, where muscles in one part of the body are weaker than in others. Studies have found that about a third of polio survivors have muscle imbalances that cause scoliosis: Their spines are being pulled to one side, because muscles on the other side are too weak to keep the spine straight. For example, if the spine is pulled to the left, a C-shaped curve is created that makes the body bend to the right and can cause muscle pain. For example, people with a curve to the right constantly use their left back, hip, and neck muscles to pull themselves to the left so that they appear straight. Having muscles continually turned on in this way is called "bracing," and it causes muscle pain.

Some polio survivors are imbalanced in another way. They have always had atrophy of muscles in one upper leg and buttock, making it smaller than the other and causing their upper bodies to tilt to the smaller side when they're seated. To appear straight, they brace muscles on the opposite side of their bodies, again causing muscle pain.

Other polio survivors have one shoulder that droops because of muscle paralysis and have learned to use their neck muscles to lift and hold the drooping shoulder in place so that it appears even with the other. Years of lifting and bracing that shoulder cause muscles to go into spasm and trigger shoulder, neck, and headache pain.

WEAKNESS, SUBSTITUTION, AND OVERUSE

Many polio survivors have learned to walk and function despite widespread muscle weakness by "substituting" stronger muscles for weaker ones. Orthopedist Jacqueline Perry found that polio survivors compensate for lower leg muscle weakness by substituting and overusing their upper leg and hip muscles. Polio survivors with foot drop will substitute their hip and lower back muscles to lift their upper leg and allow their foot to clear the ground, which causes hip and low back pain. Those with quadriceps weakness rely on their butt muscles pulling their upper leg backward and thereby lock the knee. This puts incredible strain on the knee, stretching the ligaments and causing knee pain and recurvatum, or "back knee," in which the knee joint actually does bend backward. Keep in mind that the muscles serving as substitutes were themselves weakened by the poliovirus and can't do double duty without also getting weaker over time. The weakening of substituted muscles and the added physical overuse-abuse of joints causes many small tears in tendons, ligaments, and joint cartilage. This can lead to tendinitis and bursitis, inflammation of the tendons and the bursa, the sac that cushions the joints.

Substitution also occurs above the waist. Polio survivors with weak hand and lower arm muscles will substitute their shoulder and upper back muscles in order to move their hands. This causes chronic overuse of shoulder muscles and triggers upper arm, shoulder, upper back, and neck muscle pain. Substitution and overuse trigger tendinitis and bursitis in the shoulder, what we call "post-polio shoulder."

Then there's the "upward mobility" substitution effect. PPS researcher Mary Klein found that polio survivors who have weakness of the legs develop shoulder pain, because they overuse their arms pushing themselves up from chairs. Forcing the hands backward to help stand up from sitting also explains why polio survivors, even those who haven't used canes or crutches, have more carpal tunnel syndrome—hand numbness and tingling caused by compression of the nerves that pass through the wrist into the hand—than do those with no history of polio. And of course, years of leaning on canes and crutches also causes carpal tunnel syndrome and pain in the hands, wrists, arms, and shoulders.

SPASTICITY AND INCREASED MUSCLE TONE

It isn't just new weakness and overuse that cause muscles to contract, go into spasm, and hurt. Sometimes the brain itself is unable to tell muscles to relax. In those with spinal cord injury and multiple sclerosis, the brain is disconnected from the spine and unable to tell muscles to turn off. When left to their own devices, spinal cord motor neurons do what they're supposed to do—make muscles contract. This causes spasticity, in which a muscle contracts to stop the joint to which it's attached from moving. David Bodian thought that poliovirus damage to the muscle relaxation neurons in the brain stem reticular formation may have been responsible for intense muscle contractions that caused the severe neck and back pain that Dee described accompanying her polio attack. Since reticular formation neurons remain damaged in adult polio survivors—damage that may increase with age—polio survivors' muscles may spasm more easily, spasm more intensely, and stay in spasm longer because the brain can't tell them to relax.

Another cause of muscle pain is a continuous increase in muscle tone, when a muscle shortens as it gets ready to contract. In those with cerebral palsy and after a stroke, there is damage to the motor neurons in the cortex of the brain, where the signal to turn a muscle on and off originates. This damage produces a constant increase in muscle tone that allows muscles to contract more easily and go into spasm. David Bodian found poliovirus damage to the motor neurons in the cortex, but this damage was thought to be hidden by the death of spinal cord motor neurons and is probably unrelated to muscle spasm in acute polio or PPS.

However, there is another cause of increased muscle tone in polio survivors: emotional stress. A mechanism has developed in all animals so that when they're under stress, the brain automatically shortens muscles to allow them to contract more quickly and forcefully, so that they can fight or take flight from an attacker: the "fight or flight" response. So it makes sense that our

Surveys found that emotional stress and anxiety are among the most common triggers of muscle pain, and that polio survivors whose pain was triggered by stress had more Type A behaviors. It's also no surprise that our Survey found anxiety, stress, and Type A behavior also triggered headaches, and that emotional stress was the number one cause of neck and back pain.

A Quick Fix for Pain?

In chapter 16 I'll talk in detail about ways to manage post-polio pain, which will involve changes in lifestyle, posture, and maybe using braces and assistive devices. Unfortunately, some polio survivors don't want to change or to use devices that make them look "more disabled," so they search for a quick pain fix. You can always find a doctor who will promise pain relief, but you need to be very cautious. Many doctors will explain polio survivors' back pain by saying they have herniated or bulging discs, or "pinched" nerves, adding that back surgery is the cure. And it's true that pain and numbness, especially if they travel down an arm or leg, can be caused by a herniated disc. But as much as 40 percent of the general population has herniated discs—and report no symptoms at all. What's more, studies have shown that about 99 percent of all back surgeries are unnecessary. In twenty years we have not once recommended that a post-polio patient have back surgery to treat pain.

Other doctors will tell you that polio survivors' pain can be stopped by injecting a local anesthetic into a muscle spasm (a trigger point injection) or cortisone around the spinal cord (an epidural block). However, these injections don't provide a permanent fix for chronic pain—and they may not even provide a quick fix. Botulism toxin, Botox, is also being suggested as a treatment for chronic muscle spasm. Botox paralyzes a muscle for about six months. But of all people, polio survivors need to exercise extreme caution before they voluntarily agree to have more of their muscles even temporarily paralyzed. You need to try all other treatments for pain before you let anyone inject your muscles or spine, or cut you up. We have had patients with disabling back pain come to The Post-Polio Institute as their last resort before surgery, or before having a *second* back surgery after the first didn't cure their pain. It was a change in lifestyle, using braces, crutches, and assistive devices—or in two cases just a change in posture—that "cured" their pain and made surgery unnecessary.

HANDS-ON THERAPY

The first professional you should see to evaluate pain is a physiatrist, a specialist in rehabilitation medicine, who can evaluate the possible causes for your pain and make treatment recommendations. The first treatment recommendation will likely be to send you to a physical therapist, hopefully one with lots of experience treating both PPS and chronic pain. Some physical therapists can do a special deep massage, called fibrositis massage or myofascial release, to physically separate the muscle fibers that are in spasm, lengthening and temporarily relaxing the muscle. And ultrasound, the deep heating of muscles using sound waves (done only with a prescription by a PT), can be helpful. But if heat is helpful, you can warm your muscles for free by taking a hot bath or shower and using a heating pad at home. (As I'll discuss in chapter 13, it's crucial that you keep your muscles warm, since polio survivors get cold very easily, and cold triggers muscle spasm.) But be careful. Too many physical therapists use the "shake and bake" method: gentle massage after your muscles have been heated by hot packs or ultrasound. Although massage and heat can relax muscle spasms and make you feel better for a few hours, if you don't find and stop the spasm trigger, your pain will return.

Once spasms start to relax, a home stretching program is an indispensable companion to physical therapy to keep spasms turned off. Your PT needs to help you find a few stretches that are specific for the muscles in spasm, not give you many repetitions of ten different stretches that you do only in the morning. Only a handful of stretches will be necessary to loosen up in the morning and just before bed. But it's important to find a very few specific stretches that you can do frequently throughout the day to turn off muscles that are tightening up and keep them relaxed.

A treatment I find very helpful is EMG or muscle biofeedback, which can quickly teach you how to recognize that you're overusing muscles, which muscles are tightening up, and how to turn them off, as well as teaching the "painless posture" that I'll discuss in chapter 16. Small self-adhesive electrodes are placed on painful muscles and are plugged into an electronic device the size of a transistor radio. As you go through the day, the biofeedback unit beeps when you're overusing muscles, your muscles get tight, or your posture is slipping. The beeping reminds you to relax muscles and get back into painless posture.

PRESCRIPTION FOR PAIN?

Sometimes, when you've tried absolutely everything else, you may need some extra help turning off muscle spasms and treating pain. There are over-the-counter pain medications such as aspirin, acetaminophen, and the many variations on ibuprofen, a nonsteroidal anti-inflammatory drug (NSAID). Those who experience stomach burning with ibuprofen may be able to use the less irritating anti-inflammatory drugs Celebrex and Vioxx, which are available only by prescription. NSAIDs are the only medications frequently recommended for pain at The Post-Polio Institute, but are suggested only after polio survivors have done everything else they can to manage pain.

Only under extraordinary circumstances—injury, surgery, and severe weakness that prevents polio survivors from frequent stretching on their own—are other medications considered to treat muscle spasm pain. Muscle relaxants such as Valium, baclofen, and Flexeril are very effective in treating severe muscle spasms. And Fiorinal, Ultram, and Tylenol with codeine, as well as big-league narcotics like OxyContin and morphine, are powerful pain medications. However all of these drugs cause sedation—not a good thing for polio survivors with fatigue. If you ever use a medication to treat muscle spasms or pain, take it only for a few weeks, until the pain trigger can be turned off through physical therapy, heat, stretching, biofeedback, and learning painless posture. We use these medications exceedingly rarely. There are only three Post-Polio Institute patients for whom these medications are prescribed. For the overwhelming majority of polio survivors self-care, and not medication, is the prescription for pain.

STOPPING SURGICAL SCREAMING

Still, there is one situation where polio survivors must have pain medication: when they have surgery. In our 2000 International Survey of 195 polio survivors who had undergone surgery, 20 percent reported severe and sometimes uncontrollable pain afterward. Why is surgery an occasion for giving polio survivors whatever pain medication they need for however long they need it? Because polio survivors hurt more than other people do.

One of the first things polio survivors told us back in 1982 was that they were exquisitely sensitive to pain. We measured pain sensitivity in our first laboratory study that also looked at the effects of cold on polio survivors. We applied electrical stimuli of varying strengths (yes, we're talking electric shocks here) to the hands of polio survivors and people without disabilities and discovered that polio survivors were *twice* as sensitive to pain.

Why would polio survivors be more sensitive to pain? David Bodian had the answer to this question fifty years ago. He found that the poliovirus killed the neurons in the brain and spinal cord that (as was discovered in the 1970s) make the neurochemicals endorphin and enkephalin, the body's own morphine. So polio survivors are less able to "medicate" themselves from within for pain, as is seen in this survivor's experience after stomach surgery:

The morphine concoction didn't cover it. There was only pain—pain to the furthest reaches of consciousness. No other self exists there. I was pain.

MIA, CLASS OF '54

So if you are injured, break a bone, tear some ligaments, or have dental work or surgery of any kind, remember the Post-Polio Precept we call "The Rule of 2" for pain:

POLIO SURVIVORS NEED TWO TIMES THE DOSE OF PAIN MEDICATION FOR TWO TIMES AS LONG AS NON-POLIO SURVIVORS.

Since polio survivors are typically extremely stoic, it is our experience that they neither abuse nor become dependent upon pain medication. In fact, it's often difficult to get polio survivors even to ask for pain meds, because they don't want to "depend" on pills and because they think they should "tough it out." Polio survivors should never be forced to tough out traumatic or post-op pain.

ARE MAGNETS ATTRACTIVE FOR PAIN?

Several years ago, polio survivors were studied to determine if magnets would reduce pain. Researcher Carlos Vallbona identified places on survivors' bodies that hurt. He then caused more pain "by firm application of a blunt object" to the area, asking subjects to rate pain on a scale from zero to ten. Pain was on average rated as nine. Then either a magnetic pad or an identical nonmagnetic pad was placed over the painful area for forty-five minutes and the blunt object was again pressed into the skin. Subjects wearing the magnet rated their pain a four on average, while those wearing the nonmagnetic pad rated it an eight.

Vallbona's double-blind, placebo-controlled study is an example of the gold standard of research. Unfortunately, the media and magnet manufacturers immediately reported that magnets were the "cure for post-polio pain." The problem is that pushing a blunt object into the skin is not the same as the day-to-day back, neck, muscle, or joint pain experienced by polio survivors. Without another study we can't know if magnets can decrease, let alone cure, polio survivors' pain. A 2000 study reported in the *Journal of the American Medical Association* found that wearing a magnet or an identical-looking nonmagnetic pad produced no significant relief in patients with low back pain. But even if magnets are someday found to decrease pain, polio survivors shouldn't think they can run themselves ragged, apply magnets, and everything will be fine. Please remember this important Post-Polio Precept:

TREAT THE CAUSE OF PPS, NOT THE SYMPTOM.

Pain is an indication that damage is being done to the body. When polio survivors relax muscles, develop painless posture, and use needed assistive devices, their pain can virtually disappear. When patients returning to The Post-Polio Institute tell us that pain has returned, it's a sign that they've fallen off the wagon in terms of taking care of themselves. Masking pain—with magnets or morphine—is not an appropriate treatment for pain or for *any* symptom and just makes PPS worse. This is particularly true for the most common post-polio symptom, which we'll turn to next.

CHAPTER 11

Brain Brownout

Have you ever been so exhausted that eating a meal, let alone cooking it, simply wasn't possible? Have you been so pooped that you could only sit looking down at the rug, watching for it to move? Have you ever been so wiped that you sit down, for just a minute, and wake up three hours later? Have you been so worn out that you're listening to someone speak and can't put the words they're saying together into a sentence? Have you ever been so weary that you couldn't think of the words *you* want to say? Have you been so tired that you go from one room to another to get something and forget what you've gone for once you arrive? That's *my* post-polio fatigue.

MOLLY, CLASS OF '48

Fatigue. Overwhelming, incapacitating, oh-God-don't-let-me-fall-asleep-at-the-wheel-again-and-get-me-home-into-bed fatigue.

Fatigue is the most commonly reported and most disabling PPS symptom. In our Surveys more than 90 percent of polio survivors reported new or increased fatigue, 40 percent reported fatigue significantly interfered with work, and a quarter reported fatigue interfered with their ability to care for themselves. Just over 90 percent of polio survivors in the 1985 Survey reported that fatigue was triggered by physical overexertion, while 60 percent reported that fatigue was triggered by emotional stress. Importantly, polio survivors distinguish between physical tiredness—a leaden feeling that they relate to muscle weakness—and fatigue of that most important muscle, the brain. Our 1990 Survey asked 373 polio survivors and 146 people without disabilities about symptoms of fatigue and their triggers. More than 70 percent of polio survivors reported that fatigue was associated with difficulty paying attention, concentrating, remembering, thinking clearly, finding the word they wanted to say, and staying awake during the day. More than three-quarters reported moderate to severe difficulty with these brain functions.

It was clear to us as far back as 1985 that polio survivors' problems with attention, memory, thinking, and staying awake could not be explained by poliovirus damage to motor neurons in the spinal cord. Motor neurons don't think or pay attention. Motor neurons activate muscles, they don't activate the brain. It was brain fatigue that prompted us to look at research from the 1940s to see if the poliovirus did do damage above the spinal cord.

Bodian and the Brain

As you already know from chapter 3, David Bodian found that the main event of poliovirus infection was an inflammation of the brain, a polioencephalitis, whether or not the virus got into the spinal cord. In every case of polio he studied, paralytic or "nonparalytic," Bodian saw a consistent pattern of damage to neurons in the brain stem, especially in the reticular formation that sends signals upward through your brain to activate the cortex, which keeps you awake and focuses your attention. As poliovirus itself traveled upward within the brain, brain-activating neurons in addition to those in the reticular formation were attacked, including the hypothalamus, the brain's automatic control center that activates your cortex directly and triggers release of the brain-activating hormone ACTH; the thalamus, the central relay station for information being sent up to the brain; and the basal ganglia, responsible for controlling movement as well as turning on your cortex. Not content to stop there, the poliovirus also killed the neurons that produce dopamine, the single most important neurochemical for activating your brain.

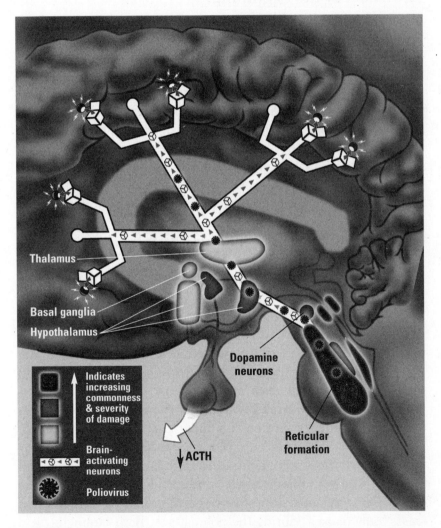

POLIOVIRUS DAMAGE TO THE BRAIN-ACTIVATING SYSTEM

Given widespread damage by the poliovirus to the entirety of the brain's activating system, you might expect that polio survivors shouldn't have had to wait forty years to experience trouble turning on their brains, staying awake, and focusing attention. And you would be right.

Brownout at the Beginning

During the epidemics there were reports of brain deactivation from the first days of the poliovirus attack. Some polio patients were described as lethargic, drowsy, sleeping constantly, and being difficult to awaken. Others were even in a coma, the ultimate result of failure of the brain's activating system.

In B. E. Holmgren's study of Swedish polio patients, at least one-third, whether they had paralytic or "nonparalytic" polio, had "disorientation, apathy, and pronounced sleep disorder." These symptoms of brain deactivation were associated with abnormal slowing of polio patients' brain waves as measured using an EEG, or electroencephalograph.

In 1947 psychologist Edith Meyer described American polio survivors ranging in age from eighteen months to fourteen years old. For three years Meyer followed these children's performance in school and measured their mental abilities. She discovered that "a high percentage of children clinically recovered from poliomyelitis insofar as motor disability is concerned, had qualitative difficulties in mental functioning which, as a rule, do not appear in the conventional type of intelligence test." Through special psychological tests, or merely by observing their performance in school, Meyer found that the children had "fatigability and fleeting attention" for months after the polio attack. When tested, she discovered that they indeed had short attention spans, difficulty concentrating, and poor memory for visual designs. These problems were "present in cases in which the medical history notes drowsiness, severe headache, and, in some cases, only nausea" during the polio attack. Both Holmgren and Meyer found that even children who had "nonparalytic" polio, who had no paralysis or even weakness, had symptoms of poliovirus damage to the brain-activating system.

But here we find another Polio Paradox. If polio survivors had the equivalent of what today could be diagnosed as attention deficit disorder, how is it that they did so well in school, went on to college, and became teachers, lawyers, chief executives of international corporations, members of parliaments and U.S. Congress, a Supreme Court justice, and an American president? And why has it taken polio survivors forty years to again report "fatigability and fleeting attention"?

We can only speculate, since today's technology was not available in the 1950s to study the brains of young polio survivors. But it's likely that polio survivors' fatigue and fleeting attention improved for the same reasons that they were able to recover muscle strength: Damaged brain neurons that survived the poliovirus onslaught may have compensated for the death of their compatriots by sending out new sprouts. Remaining, damaged neurons were pressed to release more brain-activating neurochemicals, like ACTH and dopamine, to make up for the chemicals that were no longer being produced when other brain-activating neurons died.

Regardless of the way in which brain-activating neurons recovered and allowed polio survivors to have possibly better-than-normal brain functioning for so many years, those recovery mechanisms seem to be failing in midlife, causing symptoms similar to those seen right after the polio attack. Today we not only can measure attention and concentration with psychological tests, but also have new technology that has allowed us to measure brain waves, record brain-activating chemicals, and even "look" at the post-polio brain to help us understand the cause of, and help identify treatments for, post-polio brain fatigue.

Attention!

One technology that hasn't changed much since the 1940s is the psychological tests that measure how well you pay attention, concentrate, remember, and think. We've done several studies of polio survivors using psychological tests. In the first we carefully selected our most severely fatigued post-polio patients and compared them to polio survivors with little or no fatigue. During a grueling three-hour session we tested polio survivors' attention, concentration, memory, and thinking ability. During those three hours, attention tests were given at one-hour intervals. When polio survivors with severe fatigue began taking the attention tests, they reported that their fatigue was "moderate" and made many errors. By the fourth time they took the tests, even though they reported that their fatigue was now severe, they made fewer errors than at the first try—but their scores on the tests were still not normal as compared to the general population. Polio survivors with little or no fatigue made few mistakes on the attention tests, and their scores were normal to begin with. Scores got better each time they took the tests, and their fatigue after three hours was merely mild.

Polio survivors with severe fatigue took up to two-thirds more time to complete the attention tests than did those without fatigue. But by taking extra time, fatigued polio survivors performed nearly as well as those without fatigue. So if polio survivors with fatigue and difficulty focusing attention can stick with a task, such as balancing the checkbook, they won't make many more mistakes than would anyone else . . . if, that is, they can stay awake while they're doing it.

Across all the studies we've conducted, nearly all polio survivors—regardless of their level of fatigue—made more mistakes than those with no history of polio on the most difficult attention tests, tests that demand the kind of concentration required if you're going to drive through Manhattan at rush hour. On easier attention tests, twice as many fatigued polio survivors had problems with attention as compared to polio survivors with little or no fatigue. These findings suggest, as David Bodian saw fifty years ago, that the brain-activating system is damaged in all polio survivors. Still that damage is more severe in polio survivors who report fatigue, as evidenced by their having more difficulty focusing attention even on simple tasks.

Fortunately, despite the fact that nearly 85 percent of polio survivors reported memory problems and 70 percent reported difficulty thinking clearly on our 1990 Survey, even severely fatigued polio survivors had no trouble at all on tests where they had to remember and repeat information they'd read or was read to them, or on tests of thinking ability. This means that the problems polio survivors report with memory and thinking are due to difficulty getting information into their brains, not difficulty storing the information or processing it once it's inside. So please note: Difficulty focusing attention, memory lapses, and thinking difficulties do not mean you have Alzheimer's disease. Actually, there is some evidence that polio survivors are less likely to develop Alzheimer's, evidence I'll discuss in chapter 18.

My Kingdom for a Map!

Another interesting finding came from our laboratory and from neuropsychologist D. L. Freidenberg. We both found that polio survivors, whether they have fatigue or not, have difficulty with visual memory—for example, reproducing a drawing they've been shown. This is exactly the "poor memory for designs" that Edith Meyer found when she tested her post-polio children back in the 1940s.

It's not clear why polio survivors we tested have poor visual memory. David Bodian showed us that the poliovirus did not affect two areas of the brain required for storing memories, the hippocampus and the cortex. Perhaps polio survivors' brains are less able to pay attention to images and pictures, information processed by the right side of the brain. It makes sense that polio survivors would have more trouble with the brain's right side, since it works to activate the brain in concert with the brain-activating system, which we know is damaged by the poliovirus.

Regardless of the mechanism, poor visual memory does explain why so many polio survivors tell us they always feel lost—why they have such difficulty finding their way while driving, for instance, unless they're following explicit written instructions. Apparently, poor visual memory prevents polio survivors from keeping a map in their heads of where they've been and where they're going:

> My sense of direction: It's as bad as they come. It's a curse. I can't find my way anywhere or back again, which is worse, even when shown patiently and in great detail, I can't do it. Once, when I tried to drive myself to Palm Springs, I became so hopelessly lost that I spent eight hours on the freeways.
>
> MIA, CLASS OF '54

When I told Mia that her "curse" was just another "gift" left behind by the poliovirus, she said, "I'm so relieved. I thought there was something terribly wrong with me." And that's how polio survivors usually react when they discover that they don't have Alzheimer's disease, and that there's a physical reason why they're having trouble upstairs. Yes, polio survivors have damage to their brains, but they are by no means brain damaged. Our 1985 Survey found that polio survivors have more years of education on average than do individuals with or without disabilities, and typically became superachievers: teachers, lawyers, scientists, political and business leaders—even actors. If this level of achievement is the result of brain damage, then everyone should have a little of it (plus a very good map)!

Seeing Spots

One technology that wasn't available during the polio epidemics is MRI, magnetic resonance imaging. We have used MRI to look for evidence of the poliovirus damage David Bodian saw in the brain-activating system. In our first study 90 percent of the dozen polio survivors we imaged had small areas of "hyperintense signal," which look like white spots on MRI. These spots were seen among the gray neurons in the reticular formation and basal ganglia, which were known to have been killed by the poliovirus, as well as in the "white matter," the brain's myelin-covered neurons, the "insulated wires" that connect the brain activating system to the rest of the brain.

In a second study we used MRI to image the brains of twenty-two polio survivors, this time separating them into those with and without fatigue. White spots were seen among the same gray and white neurons in 55 percent of the polio survivors with fatigue but were not seen in a single survivor without fatigue. What's more, the presence of white spots was related to polio survivors' reports of difficulty with attention, concentration, memory, thinking clearly, and mind wandering.

What are these spots? They're most likely the tombstones of gray brain-activating system neurons killed by the poliovirus. The neurons were replaced by glia, the cells that act as the "scaffolding" for brain neurons, which show up as white spots on MRI.

Then why did we find white spots among myelinated neurons that are not attacked by the poliovirus? David Bodian had answers for that, too. He thought that brain tissue might be damaged by the passage of huge amounts of poliovirus moving from the blood into the brain, possibly leaving spaces in the brain around blood vessels that fill with fluid, which show up white on MRI. Poliovirus definitely travels inside myelinated neurons all the way to the top of the brain, killing motor neurons in the cortex itself. When neurons die, their myelinated axons disintegrate and leave a space into which glia can grow or fluid can flow, which will show up as white spots. White spots on MRI among myelinated neurons have been associated with attention problems in patients with chronic fatigue syndrome and multiple sclerosis. However, the spots we saw in polio survivors are much smaller in size and number than those seen in multiple sclerosis, and a radiologist should not confuse polio survivors' spots with the plaques of MS.

You may well ask why we saw spots only in the reticular formation, in the basal ganglia, and among myelinated neurons and not in other areas attacked by the poliovirus. The explanation again comes from David Bodian. Actually, it's surprising that we were able to see spots at all. Even in polio patients who died because the reticular formation was severely damaged, Bodian found that poliovirus damage was "heavily peppered" throughout the brain stem, rather than being "composed of large discrete areas of destruction." What's more, he found that only in "a few instances" were "areas of complete neuronal destruction" seen that were as large as one millimeter in diameter. Since MRI can only image sections of the brain that are one millimeter or bigger, white spots will only be seen in polio survivors who had many neurons damaged in a specific area. This may be why we only saw spots in polio survivors with fatigue—fatigue that resulted from a relatively large amount of brain-activating system damage in one place.

Polio survivors' problems with attention and white spots on MRI were the first evidence for our notion that brain fatigue is related to damage the poliovirus did to the brain. We continued our studies using other techniques, hoping to uncover more effects of poliovirus damage to the brain-activating system.

Chemical Catnap

Another technology that wasn't available in the 1940s was the ability to measure the hormones produced by the brain. Truth be told, few of the hormones produced by the brain were even known about fifty years ago. Bodian and other researchers found that the poliovirus damaged the front, back, and sides of the hypothalamus, which produces hormones that regulate the body's internal environment and its response to stress. One area of the hypothalamus the poliovirus damaged was the part that releases the hormone CRH. When you're under emotional or physical stress, CRH is released and tells your pituitary gland to release another hormone, ACTH, into your blood. ACTH then travels to the adrenal glands that sit on top of your kidneys and tells them to release cortisol, the body's main antistress hormone.

What's important about this chain of chemical events? Both

CRH and ACTH have been found to be brain-activating chemicals. Injecting ACTH into anyone speeds up brain waves, improves alertness, increases attention, and causes a significant reduction in fatigue. Too little CRH and ACTH might cause symptoms of brain fatigue, especially when polio survivors are under stress. And our patients' stress response was something we wanted to know more about, since 60 percent of polio survivors in our 1985 Survey reported that fatigue was triggered or increased by emotional stress.

So we did two studies to measure ACTH in the blood of polio survivors using the most gentle stress that can cause a release of ACTH: an overnight fast. In polio survivors reporting little or no fatigue ACTH increased with the fast, as it should. But there was no increase in ACTH in polio survivors reporting severe daily fatigue. The more difficulty with memory, word finding, and staying awake during the day, polio survivors reported, the less ACTH they released. In polio survivors who had brain fatigue, it seemed that either the brain didn't know it was under stress, or it couldn't respond to stress with an increase in ACTH. It appears that poliovirus damage to one part of hypothalamus results in the reduced release of ACTH, which would be a special problem for polio survivors under emotional or physical stress—the very time when they would need the extra boost this brain-activating chemical would provide.

Catching a Slow Wave

So far it looks like the poliovirus has done some dirty deeds north of the spinal cord, too. Polio survivors have fatigue, have trouble focusing attention, and don't make a chemical they need to turn on the brain when it's under stress. We even have pictures of poliovirus damage to brain-activating neurons. But there is a way to actually show that post-polio brain neurons have been deactivated: measuring brain waves.

Remember that Holmgren found brain waves slowing in children who were disorientated and apathetic right after they had

polio. We measured brain waves in middle-aged polio survivors
and found that the more fatigue they reported, the slower the
brain waves on the *right* side of their brains. Aha! Remember
that the right side of the brain is thought to activate the entire
brain, and that polio survivors have trouble with visual memory,
which is thought to be controlled by the right side of the brain.
A damaged brain-activating system may slow the right side of the
brain—and thereby slow the entire brain—as well as make it difficult for Mia to find her way to Palm Springs.

When we measured polio survivors' brain waves, we also
measured another hormone, prolactin, because the more prolactin there is in the blood, the less dopamine is being made by
the brain. The more prolactin we found in the blood (and therefore the less dopamine in the brain), the more fatigue polio survivors reported, and the slower their brain waves. The possibility
that a shortage of brain dopamine is related to polio survivors'
fatigue suggests some fascinating parallels between polio and
Parkinson's disease that may help explain why post-polio brain
fatigue occurs decades after the poliovirus attack.

Polio–Parkinson's Parallels

Parkinson's disease, with its characteristic tremors and rigidity, is
also associated with difficulty focusing attention and fatigue.
Nearly half of Parkinsonians in one study reported "excessive
fatigue," while almost one-third in another study said that fatigue
was their "most disabling symptom." As a matter of fact, one of
the first descriptions of Parkinson's disease could serve as a definition of post-polio brain fatigue: "a diminution of voluntary
attention . . . and the capacity for effort and work, with significant and objective fatigability, and a slight diminution of
memory."

It is the failure and death of dopamine neurons in midlife,
possibly in addition to the death of some number of dopamine
neurons early in life, that is thought to be responsible for the
appearance of Parkinson's symptoms. So, too, as polio survivors

reach midlife, brain fatigue symptoms may appear as a result of the failure and death of some remaining polio-damaged brain-activating system neurons—especially dopamine neurons—in addition to those killed during the poliovirus attack. Why "especially" dopamine neurons? By the time everyone reaches fifty, they have lost about one-third of the dopamine neurons in their brains. What's worse, the remaining neurons begin to appear shriveled, and the protein that makes dopamine has decreased by at least 70 percent. Since polio survivors lost dopamine neurons during the poliovirus attack, it would just be a matter of time before aging alone could lead to the loss of enough dopamine neurons and cause a brain activation brownout.

A Parkinson's–Polio Paradox

If polio patients had damage to their dopamine neurons, why didn't they develop the tremor and rigidity that are characteristic of Parkinson's disease during the polio attack? This question was asked in 1948 by H. W. Magoun, the researcher who discovered that the reticular formation is the heart of the brain-activating system. Magoun explained what he himself called a paradox by referring to David Bodian's research. Magoun concluded that if poliovirus damage to dopamine neurons is severe, "injury to the lower brain stem reticular formation is intense, some of the vital centers are destroyed and the patient does not survive." Patients with intense injury died of "bulbar" polio, so there wasn't an opportunity for tremor and rigidity to be seen. However, Magoun added that if reticular formation injury is less severe, it would be "below the threshold necessary" for Parkinson's symptoms to be seen, since 70 percent of dopamine neurons must be killed for tremor and rigidity to appear. The notion that severe damage to the dopamine-producing neurons is accompanied by fatal damage to the reticular formation is supported by the observation that nearly all of the reported cases of polio in which Parkinson's tremor and rigidity did appear were rapidly fatal.

Over the years, we have seen no greater number of polio survivors with tremor and rigidity among our patients than would be seen in the general population. But we have noted that one Parkinson's symptom is common among polio survivors.

Let Me Say This About That

Of all the symptoms of brain fatigue that polio survivors report, there was one we never expected: word-finding difficulty. In the 1990 Survey more than three-quarters of polio survivors told us they had difficulty "thinking of words I want to say," with more than one-third reporting frequent, moderate to severe difficulty finding words. The more severe the fatigue polio survivors reported and the greater their difficulty focusing attention, the greater the word-finding difficulty.

What is word-finding difficulty? Parkinson's patients describe it as the "tip-of-the-tongue" experience; they know the word they want to say but can't get it out. The "lost words" are usually the names of familiar objects or familiar people—sometimes even family members! We tested polio survivors' ability to find words by asking them to name as many animals as they could in one minute. (Give this a try if you'd like before reading on.)

Polio survivors with fatigue could name only seventeen animals on average, which is exactly the number of animals that Parkinson's disease patients can name. The normal number is at least eighteen. What's more, the fewer animals polio survivors could name, the higher their prolactin (and therefore the lower their brain dopamine) and the worse they scored on tests of attention. So word-finding difficulty is yet another piece of evidence linking brain fatigue in polio survivors with trouble focusing attention and poliovirus damage to the brain-activating system, especially to the loss of dopamine neurons.

If dopamine is the main brain-activating neurochemical and polio survivors have too little of it, we wondered in 1995 if a drug that replaced dopamine would reduce the symptoms of post-polio fatigue, including difficulty with word finding and attention.

A Drug Treatment for Fatigue?

Several drugs affect the amount of dopamine that is available in the brain. However, we didn't want to use amphetamines or Ritalin, since they would "squeeze" poliovirus-damaged neurons and force them to release dopamine. We also didn't want to depend on the remaining, already overworked poliovirus-damaged neurons to make dopamine. So we rejected monoamine oxidase inhibitors, MAOIs, such as deprenyl, which prevent the breakdown of dopamine that is already released by neurons. We were left with L-Dopa, which is converted to dopamine in the brain, and bromocriptine, which bypasses dopamine neurons entirely and directly stimulates dopamine receptors on brain-activating system neurons. We chose to do an end run and tested bromocriptine.

We looked at the records of all the patients who had successfully completed treatment with us before 1995 and eliminated those who had potential causes for fatigue other than PPS, such as depression, a slow thyroid, anemia, breathing or sleeping difficulties, or diabetes. Of the remaining patients, only 10 percent continued to report at least moderate daily fatigue after treatment. Five patients agreed to be in the study, and they took a placebo and then increasing doses of bromocriptine for twenty-eight days as they completed daily logs rating all their brain fatigue symptoms.

Three patients reported a noticeable reduction in fatigue symptoms on bromocriptine as compared to placebo, saying that they "felt awake" and "had a clear head" for the first time in years. The higher the dose of bromocriptine, the lower their daily difficulty with attention, word finding, mind wandering, concentration, memory, and thinking clearly. Fatigue upon awakening decreased by just over 50 percent. These patients had more poliovirus damage to their brain-activating systems, as shown by their having more than twice as many white spots on MRIs, abnormally low scores on tests of attention, no increase in ACTH after an overnight fast, and nearly twice as much prolactin as the two patients who did not respond to bromocriptine.

Do these results mean that bromocriptine is the treatment of choice for post-polio fatigue? Absolutely not. The study's most important finding was that almost 90 percent of the polio survivors we had treated were not eligible for the drug trial since their daily fatigue was less than moderate after they had applied all the symptom management techniques that I'll discuss in chapter 16. You'll see that the treatment of choice for brain fatigue—for all PPS—is not bromocriptine but The Golden Rule. Only after all symptom management techniques are consistently applied should bromocriptine even be considered. As a matter of fact, we have not given bromocriptine to one patient since the study ended, so effective is self-care in managing PPS.

Just Say No to Drugs, Again

As I've noted, drugs are not effective in treating muscle weakness, and they should only be used as last resorts for treating pain or fatigue. But there is a common drug that polio survivors use to treat fatigue without even thinking about it: caffeine. We have patients who drink four cups of coffee in the morning, swig soda all afternoon, and then down more coffee during dinner to keep themselves awake. Caffeine is a drug, and polio survivors should limit themselves to two eight-ounce cups of coffee or tea in the morning, one soda or iced tea at lunch, and have nothing with caffeine at dinner, especially if they have trouble falling asleep.

Obviously, polio survivors shouldn't be taking "pep pills"—either caffeine tablets or prescribed amphetamines—to stay awake and mask their fatigue. It's important to know that, like muscle weakness and pain, fatigue is your body's way of telling you to "sit down!"

KNOCK-OUT DROPS

It's also important to know that brain fatigue can be caused by drugs prescribed for common medical conditions. For example, antihistamines taken for allergy symptoms, tricyclic antidepressants such as Elavil, anti-anxiety medications like Valium, muscle relaxants such as Flexeril, narcotics, and high blood pressure medications (especially the beta blockers) are more sedating for polio survivors than for those who've never had polio. And of course drugs intended to be sedating—sleeping pills and intravenous and gas anesthetics—will knock out polio survivors in a trice!

You need to tell your doctor that you are easily sedated before taking any medication, and especially before you receive an anesthetic. In our 2000 Survey 237 polio survivors told us about complications they had experienced after receiving anesthesia. Far and away the biggest problem reported was being excessively sedated when they were put under. Just over half told us they were snowed after receiving a general anesthetic, and about a quarter were overly sedated when they had an endoscopy or colonoscopy, sometimes with frightening results:

> The first time I was scheduled for surgery, they gave me Valium to relax and I went to sleep. I didn't wake up for eight hours. They had to cancel the surgery. I think they were concerned.

> Each time I am put to sleep it's harder for me to awaken. At age forty-two it took two days to awaken from the general anesthetic after a hysterectomy.

> I lost the first seven days following the scope because I simply could not wake up fully. It took me weeks—probably about six weeks—to feel fully awake.

After surgery, I became aware of people talking around me, but couldn't move anything or open my eyes. I was very frightened. I thought I was dying and hearing angels. I was told I came down to the recovery room at 10 A.M. and didn't come out of the anesthetic or recovery room until 6 P.M. This was a same-day procedure and the nurses made me go home at six o'clock, even though I was not fully awake and couldn't stand by myself. They were angry with me because, if I couldn't go home, they would have had to put me in the hospital overnight and would have delayed their going home.

IN WITH THE GOOD AIR

Another finding of the 2000 Survey was that a quarter of polio survivors had difficulty breathing after receiving anesthesia, which is likely due in part to anesthetics putting reticular formation's breathing neurons to sleep. The use of curarelike drugs during major surgery, which paralyze muscles that are going to be cut and make it easier for the ventilator to fill the lungs while patients are on the table, also affects breathing. Obviously, any drug that interferes with already damaged motor neurons will prevent polio survivors from moving or even breathing for hours longer than patients who didn't have polio. Breathing difficulties are more than frightening. They can be life-threatening:

The operation was at 9 A.M. and I was told that I would be back in the ward and awake before 10. At 2 P.M. I was in intensive care and not breathing. I eventually came round at 4 P.M. but I really had to fight for every breath; each felt like it could have been my last. I had a very difficult time breathing and waking for two or three days.

When I awoke after a complete hysterectomy I vividly remember that I couldn't breathe and the silent panic that engulfed me. While nurses chatted I struggled mightily to inhale. I felt like I had fifty lead bricks on my chest. I could not even call for help. I remember the terror when I exhaled and I just couldn't start inhaling. I remember thinking how easy it would be to die for lack of the next breath. It was by sheer willpower that I forced myself to take one torturous, slow, shallow breath after another until finally a nurse came by. I was able to say "can't breathe," to her, and she helped me.

I stopped breathing in recovery. My surgeon said the anesthesiologist started yelling, "It's got to be the polio!"

Yes, it's the polio. And the bottom line for anesthesia or any medication that is sedating is a Post-Polio Precept, another "Rule of 2":

DOCTORS NEED TO DIVIDE BY TWO THE AMOUNT OF ANESTHESIA OR SEDATIVE MEDICATION GIVEN, AND POLIO SURVIVORS NEED TWO TIMES AS LONG FOR THE EFFECT OF THE MEDICATION TO WEAR OFF.

This "Rule of 2" is absolutely not intended to dictate the dose of anesthetic polio survivors receive, but merely to remind anesthesiologists that polio survivors need less anesthetic than do other patients and to start with a low dose and go up from there. As always, the dose of anesthetic must be individually adjusted for body weight and other factors, and be adequate to keep patients under during surgery. But it should not cause polio survivors to sleep for a week.

Because of polio survivors' problems with anesthesia there is another Post-Polio Precept:

POLIO SURVIVORS SHOULD NEVER HAVE SAME-DAY SURGERY.

Even applying the "Rule of 2," polio survivors may be very sedated, if not asleep, for hours after surgery. This is one of the reasons why same-day surgery—even for complicated dental procedures—is not advisable for polio survivors. Sleeping or excessively sedated polio survivors cannot be expected to return home and take care of themselves after same-day surgery, since surgical complications may go unnoticed and sedation-impaired coordination makes falling likely. Doctors should perform procedures that would usually be done in their offices—including colonoscopies and endoscopies—in the hospital and, despite HMO pressure, be prepared to admit polio survivors overnight for their own safety.

Beware the Broad Brush

With all this talk about the inevitable failure and loss of brain-activating system neurons, there may be a tendency to blame any and all new symptoms, especially fatigue, on poliovirus damage to the brain. But please remember this Post-Polio Precept:

ALL PPS—ESPECIALLY FATIGUE—ARE DIAGNOSES OF EXCLUSION!

You need to work with your doctor to rule out all other possible causes for your fatigue: a slow thyroid, anemia, daytime breathing difficulty, diabetes, depression, and especially sleep disorders. Sleep disorders are the most common and easily treatable causes of fatigue in polio survivors. So try to get a good night's sleep, come back tomorrow, and we'll talk about sleep disorders polio survivors don't even know they have.

CHAPTER 12

To Sleep, Perchance to Sleep?

I don't know what happened! I was sound asleep one moment and the next my wife is yelling and blood is running out of her nose. She screamed, "You hit me! You hit me!" I was asleep, I swear! She said my arm flew out sideways and smacked her in the face. I know I do snore. And she's been telling me for years that I stop breathing and my muscles twitch in my sleep. But why would I hit her? Please tell me it's a post-polio thing!

CHARLES, CLASS OF '48

I took this frantic phone call the day after Albert Sabin and I were on *Nightline*. Charles's wife's battered nose was the not-so-subtle clue that polio survivors, in addition to all of their other new symptoms, were also having problems during sleep. But what could have caused Charles to hit his wife in the nose while he was asleep? Was this actually "a post-polio thing"? We decided to find out.

Twitching and Jumping

In the 1985 Survey we asked polio survivors about sleeping problems, and just over half reported trouble falling asleep because their "minds are racing." Not unexpectedly, the more Type A behavior polio survivors reported, the more trouble they had turning their minds off and falling asleep. What we didn't expect were polio survivors' responses to two questions Charles prompted us to ask: "Do your muscles twitch or jump as you fall asleep?" and "Is your sleep disturbed by muscle twitching?" Remarkably, just over 60 percent reported that their muscles *did* twitch and jump during sleep, and half of those said that their sleep was disturbed by twitching. About twice as many polio survivors reported twitching in our Survey as did those who never had polio.

I shouldn't have been surprised that polio survivors had the twitches. In his 1974 biography, polio survivor William O. Douglas wrote, "I had no endurance in my legs. They tired easily, and when I exercised even mildly they would ache and twitch all night." Although our patients told us muscle twitching was more common after exercise, twitching wasn't necessarily related to overexertion. But I had no idea why polio survivors' muscles twitched. What's worse, I had no clue as to why Charles's arm flew out and clocked his wife. Could twitching become hitting?

SLEEPING SUBJECTS

To find out for ourselves what was happening during sleep, a group of our post-polio patients underwent sleep studies in 1995. Brain waves, arm and leg movements, breathing, and the amount of oxygen in the blood were measured during the night while they were supposed to be sleeping. What we found was remarkable, and included another first for polio survivors.

We found not one but four different types of twitching and jumping, including a polio survivor whose arm very easily could have flown across the bed in the middle of the night and smacked a spouse:

• **Periodic Leg Movements in Sleep.** Forty percent of the patients had periodic leg movements in sleep, PLMS, the typical form of twitching in which only leg muscles move. Only one of the patients was aware of her PLMS—and well she might be, since her leg muscle contractions were so violent that she was propelled as much as two inches off the surface of the bed.

Another patient had no idea his legs were twitching or that his brain was being awakened more than two hundred times a night by the twitches. Twitching prevented him from having any rapid eye movement (REM) sleep—the stage of sleep during which most dreaming occurs—and hardly any deep sleep, during which it's thought you get the most rest. This patient's brain spent about half the night awake. Little wonder he awoke mornings feeling like he hadn't slept:

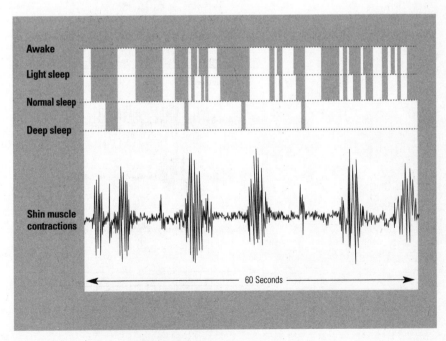

PLMS Disturbing Sleep

• **Generalized Random Myoclonus.** Almost 30 percent of the patients had what we dubbed generalized random myoclonus, GRM, a fancy way of saying that not just the legs but muscles all over the body, including toes, arms, hands—even face and chest muscles—twitch and contract randomly throughout the body throughout the night. This type of nocturnal muscle movement had never been seen before. GRM is another polio survivor first.

One patient knew all too well that her muscles were moving, since powerful contractions of her belly muscles awakened her repeatedly during the night when her body was pulled into the fetal position. A second patient had been completely unaware of moving muscles until they were noticed by her husband. She had a remarkable symphony of movements: random, rapid contractions in arms and legs, jaw and chest muscles, as well as slow, repeated grasping movements of the hands, slow flexing of the arms and wrists, and up, down, forward, and backward movements of the shoulders, as you can see:

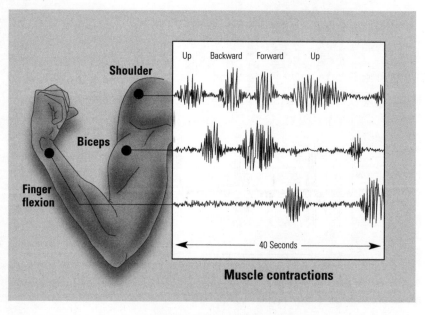

GRM DURING SLEEP

Even the toes on her right foot contracted during the night, which was remarkable since her right leg has always been totally paralyzed except for a minimal ability of the toes to move.

• **Restless Legs Syndrome Plus PLMS.** Almost 30 percent of the patients had PLMS plus restless legs syndrome. RLS is not leg muscle twitching while you're sleeping but a feeling that you *must* make your legs move. This feeling increases during the evening and often prevents sleep because people feel they must move their legs or even have to get out of bed and walk.

• **Sleep Start.** Fortunately for Charles's marriage, we found a patient whose nighttime shadowboxing was identical to his own. One patient had what's called a "sleep start," her arms forcefully flying outward from her body as she began to fall asleep. Had her husband been in the bed and his nose in range at the time she was falling asleep, he would have been in the same shape as Charles's wife. This patient knew about her sleep start, since her ballistic arm movements would prevent her from falling asleep.

Violent muscle contractions are obvious, since they wake polio survivors from sleep. Restless leg syndrome and sleep starts are also no secret, since they prevent polio survivors from falling asleep. But PLMS and GRM are sneaky. Sixty percent of the patients who had sleep studies didn't know that their muscles were twitching and jumping. This is the sneaky part—patients also didn't know that twitching prevented them from having hardly any slow-wave or REM sleep or that their brains woke up repeatedly during the night even though they were mostly unconscious. Sleeping this poorly, it makes sense that these patients reported moderate to severe daytime fatigue.

PATIENTLY SLEEPING

Because sleep problems are so common in polio survivors, we take a sleep history from patients *and* their bed partners as part of our initial evaluation. Since 1998 one-quarter of Post-Polio

Institute patients have had a sleep study recommended because they reported disturbed sleep—muscle twitching while falling asleep; waking in the middle of the night with anxiety, heart racing, choking, shortness of breath, or muscle jumping; had headaches or weren't rested upon awakening most mornings. We also recommended sleep studies if bed partners noticed snoring, twitching, or times when patients stopped breathing during sleep, or if patients' fatigue did not decrease despite successful completion of The Post-Polio Institute program and following The Golden Rule.

One-third of the patients didn't have a sleep study performed, because they didn't want to, they were afraid to spend the night in a hospital, or their medical insurance would not cover the cost. Of those who had sleep studies, one-third were found to have at least fifteen abnormal muscle movements each hour during the night (the number thought to be significant in terms of disturbing sleep). On average patients' muscles twitched nearly once every minute. The all-time twitching champ was a patient who had over seven hundred muscle movements during the night and was awakened nearly twice every minute!

WHEREFORE GRM?

Of course the "$64,000 question" is why so many polio survivors have muscle twitching, and why only polio survivors, and no one else, have movements in muscles all over the body as well as in their legs. In people with no polio history, muscle movements during sleep are thought to be caused by abnormal firing of spinal cord motor neurons and neurons in the brain—the reticular formation, thalamus, cerebellum, and basal ganglia. Given the location and severity of poliovirus damage in the spinal cord and all these brain areas, it's no wonder that a majority of polio survivors have muscles that twitch and jump at night.

The combination of nighttime twitching and basal ganglia damage is interesting because it points out other parallels between polio and Parkinson's disease: Leg muscle movements are common in Parkinson's patients. Also, both nocturnal movements and restless legs decrease when patients are given drugs that replace dopamine in the brain, such as L-Dopa, suggesting that these symptoms are related to a lack of dopamine in the brain. When our patients who had both PLMS and RLS were given Sinemet, a drug that contains L-Dopa, they had an 80 percent reduction in movements, decreased feelings of needing to move their legs, and a restful night's sleep.

But the use of drugs that replace dopamine in the brain is problematic, since they can overstimulate dopamine neurons, causing them to become less sensitive to dopamine and eventually making the drugs less effective. While dopamine-replacing drugs may be necessary to treat RLS, we have found that a very low dose of alprazolam (Xanax), an anti-anxiety and muscle-relaxing drug, taken thirty minutes before bed stops twitching and jumping (even in the patient with flailing arms). Xanax, a member of the Valium family, leaves the body quickly and doesn't cause the morning "hangover" and daytime fatigue associated with Valium and most sleeping medications. However, Xanax can affect breathing during the night, which is a concern for polio survivors. Breathing problems are another unnoticed cause of disturbed sleep in survivors that result from too little muscle movement, not too much.

To Breathe or Not to Breathe

Of The Post-Polio Institute patients who had sleep studies, nearly half were found to be breathing abnormally. We found three kinds of breathing problems during sleep; all caused abnormally low levels of oxygen in the blood that made patients' brains awaken many times during the night:

- **Central Sleep Apnea.** Ten percent of our patients had central sleep apnea (*apnea* meaning "without air"), in which the diaphragm stops moving because reticular formation neurons that should automatically tell it to contract to pull air into the lungs stop firing. On a very small scale, central sleep apnea results from the same process that caused "bulbar" polio survivors' diaphragms to stop moving for hours, days, or weeks.

• **Obstructive Sleep Apnea.** Fifteen percent of our patients had obstructive sleep apnea, in which muscles in the back of the throat become very relaxed and the tissue becomes "floppy" during sleep, closing off the throat and physically preventing air from entering the lungs.

• **Hypopnea.** A whopping 60 percent of our patients had hypopneas (meaning "low air"), where air can enter the lungs, but oxygen falls anyway because the diaphragm is not able to move enough air in and out. Hypopneas are the sneakiest of all sleep disorders because, even if someone were looking, they couldn't tell you weren't moving enough air in and out of your lungs and that blood oxygen was dropping.

On average our patients had an apnea or hypopnea every three minutes. The champs were one patient who had 160 apneas during the night, and another with more than 300 hypopneas. And remember that twitching and breathing problems are not mutually exclusive. Almost 50 percent of our patients had both. Overall, the combination of twitching and breathing problems resulted in our patients losing 60 percent of their deep sleep, and 20 percent of REM sleep. Is it any wonder that these patients would feel tired in the morning and fatigued all day long?

WHY ISN'T THERE AIR?

Sleep apnea has been seen before in polio survivors and, like abnormal movements, should have been expected. Both the reticular formation breathing neurons and the spinal cord motor neurons that actually move the diaphragm were damaged by the poliovirus. Other studies have found that both central apnea and hypopneas are up to six times more common in those who had had "bulbar" polio, despite these patients breathing normally during the day. Hypopneas have been found to occur more frequently in those who have scoliosis; the spinal curvature can reduce the size and also increases the stiffness of the chest. But the majority of our patients with apneas and hypopneas did not have "bulbar" polio or any breathing difficulty during their bouts with polio, nor do they have scoliosis or breathing problems today. So remember this Post-Polio Precept:

POLIO SURVIVORS WITHOUT SCOLIOSIS, "BULBAR" POLIO, OR BREATHING PROBLEMS—EITHER TODAY OR WHEN THEY HAD POLIO—CAN STILL HAVE SLEEP APNEA AND HYPOPNEAS.

Remember, too, that sleep disorders must be identified and treated *before* a diagnosis of PPS can be made, since the degree of sleep disturbance found in many of our patients could cause a variety of symptoms that sound just like PPS: fatigue, daytime sleepiness, difficulty with concentration and memory, decreased muscle strength, muscle pain, headache, irritability, anxiety, depression, and even decreased interest in sex.

Pumping You Up

So what's to be done about breathing problems during sleep? The simplest and most effective treatment is positive airway pressure, "PAP," where a bread-box-sized machine blows air into a mask held in place over your nose, mouth, or both by straps around your head to prevent floppy muscles from closing off the throat and to keep the lungs fully inflated. There are two kinds of PAP machines. CPAP—continuous positive airway pressure—machines blow a continuous stream of air into the lungs to keep them filled. BiPAP—bi-level positive airway pressure—machines blow air at one pressure as you're breathing in and at a much lower pressure when you breathe out. Although many patients do well with CPAP, BiPAP may be better for polio survivors, because it allows them to exhale more easily.

Some polio survivors who have hypopneas or who have very tight chest muscles may need a volume ventilator. Volume ventilators blow air into the lungs until they have been filled to a given volume, like blowing air into a balloon until it's full. Because BiPAP machines are about twice as expensive as CPAPs, and volume ventilators are about twice as expensive as BiPAPs, insurance companies are going to want you to try the cheaper machines and prove you're unable to sleep before allowing you to trade up. Make sure you and your doctor write down problems you have with various types of machines, the pressure and volume settings, and with different types of masks you try, so you can make a case for the devices you need.

Keep in mind that nighttime and daytime breathing difficulties may reveal themselves at inconvenient times, like when you're ill or are having surgery. Since polio survivors lose about 2 percent of their lung volume each year, as compared to 1 percent in people who've never had polio, any lung problem—from an upper respiratory infection to pneumonia—must be taken seriously and should be attended to by your doctor without delay. All polio survivors should have lung function tests before they have surgery and should inform their surgeon—and especially their anesthesiologist—about their polio breathing history, as well as any nighttime or daytime breathing problems, long before the morning of the operation. For polio survivors using nighttime ventilators, special arrangements must be made with the nursing staff concerning use and care of the equipment before hospital admission.

Pain Never Sleeps

Another hidden cause of disturbed sleep is pain. Research has found that sleep can be disturbed if your muscles and joints hurt. Although many polio survivors hate to hear this, the best way to prevent nighttime neck, upper back, and headache pain, as well as joint pain in your shoulders or hips, is to sleep on your back. Sleeping on your side is actually hurtful, since it puts all your weight on one bottom shoulder and hip, while the shoulder and arm on top fall down and forward, shortening your neck muscles and allowing them to spasm. It's even worse to be a stomach sleeper, because you forcefully twist your upper spine to one side and shorten your neck muscles.

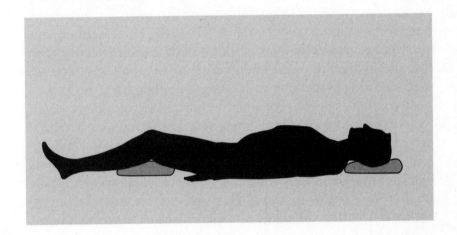

GOOD SLEEPING POSITION

One tool that might help you be comfortable sleeping on your back is a fiber-filled cervical pillow, which looks like a square doughnut. It has a fabric cradle in the center for your head and firm edges prevent your head from rolling to the side. These pillows also have a firm ridge that creates a normal C-shaped curve in your neck, keeps your head in line with your upper body, and presses on your neck muscles for a gentle, all-night massage. However, polio survivors with sleep apnea may snore and close off their throats when they lie on their backs, which makes the use of CPAP or BiPAP invaluable.

If you have pain in your lower back, a pillow under both knees can be helpful. And our patients with hip or shoulder pain get relief from an "egg crate" foam mattress cover, which gives your entire body a little cushioning to take weight off your joints.

To Sleep at All

Although pain, twitching, apneas, and especially hypopneas can be hidden causes of disturbed sleep, insomnia is all too apparent. It's no secret that polio survivors have trouble falling asleep, can wake up frequently during the night for no reason, and awaken far too early. In the 1985 Survey 50 percent of polio survivors told us they had trouble falling asleep because their "minds are racing"; and one-quarter of our patients reported early-morning awakening with difficulty falling back to sleep.

If you have these problems, the first thing you need to do is to rule out depression as their cause. Trouble falling asleep and especially waking too early are symptoms of depression. Fifteen percent of Post-Polio Institute patients have been diagnosed with a major depressive episode. While psychotherapy, and not medication, is the first line of treatment for depression, the SSRIs—selective serotonin reuptake blockers, such as Prozac, Paxil, and Zoloft—are very effective antidepressants in those who need them. However, these SSRIs can be stimulating— sometimes so stimulating that patients can't fall asleep. What's more, the SSRIs reduce REM sleep and can themselves cause frequent awakening, not exactly what polio survivors who have trouble sleeping need. The newer antidepressants, such as trazodone, Serzone, and Remeron, are equally effective at treating depression and are also sedating, so they can help you fall asleep. These drugs don't cause awakening during the night or decrease REM sleep. However, the sedating effect of these drugs can cause a morning-after hangover, with trouble waking up in addition to daytime sleepiness and fatigue.

Morning hangovers, daytime sleepiness, fatigue, and loss of REM sleep—not to mention physical and psychological dependence—are reasons that neither sedating antidepressants nor sleeping pills are appropriate treatments for insomnia. We do recommend Ambien when polio survivors have trouble falling asleep while they are getting used to using CPAP or BiPAP machines, since Ambien apparently does not reduce REM and deep sleep. But you shouldn't take sleeping pills for more than ten days, according to the drug companies, because they are habit forming and make it very difficult for you to fall asleep on your own. So what can you do if you can't fall asleep?

"SLEEP HYGIENE"

The key to beating insomnia is good "sleep hygiene," which begins from the moment you get up. It is important to schedule rest breaks during the day, just to let your body know that resting is actually a part of living. If you do nap, try what NASA has dubbed "Power Naps." Pilots took planned forty-minute rest periods during which they slept for about thirty minutes. After the nap, pilots had increased alertness and performance and relief from "significant sleepiness." Similar benefits were found in a study of healthy elderly folk. A thirty-minute nap at 1 P.M. significantly reduced afternoon sleepiness and fatigue.

But with napping, as with so many other aspects of life, there can be too much of a good thing. Longer naps can be detrimental, causing grogginess, headaches and a "sluggish" brain after awakening, which has been given the wonderful name "sleep inertia" (a body at rest tends to stay at rest). NASA Power Nap researchers discovered that deep sleep began about thirty minutes into a nap. That's how researchers determined that thirty minutes was the ideal lap length: No deep sleep, no sleep inertia.

But sleep inertia isn't napping's only detrimental effect. If you get too much sleep during the day you may not be able to fall asleep or stay asleep at night. Lack of nighttime sleep makes you more fatigued during the day, makes you nap longer, and gives you even more trouble sleeping at night. But polio survivors and others with brain activating system damage may need more than a thirty-minute nap. If thirty minutes doesn't do it for you, add fifteen minutes to your next nap. But don't sleep for more than ninety minutes or nap after 5 P.M. to prevent sleep inertia and trouble falling asleep at bedtime.

Trouble falling asleep at bedtime can also be caused by polio survivors running on an adrenaline high all day, preventing them from coming down when it's time to go to sleep. Take at least thirty minutes to wind down before bed: Do some stretching, take a hot bath, read, do a quiet meditation. If your mind is racing about your day today or what you have to do tomorrow — and tomorrow, and tomorrow — keep a pad by the bed to write down your thoughts and goals. You might want to do this just before the thirty-minute wind down. Don't have the TV or radio on as you fall asleep because the sound itself can awaken your brain. Set a daily sleep schedule and keep it all week. If you need eight hours of sleep and must get up at 7 A.M. plan to be asleep by 11 P.M. every night, including the weekends.

If you can't fall asleep or if you wake up and think you're not going to get back to sleep, get out of bed and go to another room. You can again do some gentle stretching, meditation and take some slow, deep breaths. Try reading something heavy that requires thinking (like this book), but don't pick up an engaging novel, do work or watch TV or a movie. When you feel tired, get back into bed, take some slow, deep breaths and gently drift off. If you can reset your schedule and remind your body and brain that life consists of both working *and* resting, that there is a time for being active and for being still, sleep will come on its own in time.

But when you arise in the morning after a good night's sleep, all cozy and warm, another PPS symptom makes itself known when your warm feet hit the cold tile of the bathroom floor.

CHAPTER 13

Baby, It's Cold Inside

In 1989, I started to have fatigue and burning in my right "polio" arm and lost the strength to hold a pen. I was diagnosed with PPS, had a wrist fusion to make my wrist more stable, and went on with my life, but with little use of my right hand and arm.

In 1997 I began working in an office where the temperature year-round was 59 degrees. Cold air constantly blew on my shoulders and neck. Within months, fatigue and weakness in my "good" left arm, which I thought was unaffected by the polio, became totally overwhelming. It took too much arm strength and there was too much pain to undress when I came home from work. I fell asleep in my clothes. And I wasn't the only one having trouble. Other office workers sat with coats and gloves on. My employer would not turn up the heat, no matter how much I asked, no matter how many letters my doctor wrote. I finally had to go out on disability.

For the first three months on disability I had to lie in bed under blankets almost every day to keep warm. I truly thought I would never know what being warm was again. I discovered that, because of the cold, my legs had gotten weaker, too. It was rec-ommended that I wear short braces on my legs and use a cane.

My arms and legs have never recovered. I can't lift things. I have trouble steering the car and pushing a door open. I drop glasses and can't write for more than fifteen minutes. My neck and arms and shoulders still hurt. Pain wakes me up at night. I can't walk any distance so I just got a power wheelchair. I guess this is as good as I am going to get.

MARGO, CLASS OF '53

What could have happened to Margo? How could she become overwhelmed by fatigue, permanently weakened in her arms and legs, and have constant pain just from having worked in a cold office?

This happens to be where our laboratory research on PPS began. That first polio survivor who called me twenty years ago said that his "polio" arm was always colder than his other arm. The first polio survivor we studied said her polio-affected foot turned purple when she was in a room that was comfortably cool to everyone else. I was shocked and worried when she removed her sock to reveal a reddish purple calf and a deep purple foot. I was afraid she had a blood clot, maybe even a clogged artery. But her veins were clear, and she had bounding pulses in both feet. The real shock came when I placed an electronic thermometer on her skin. The room temperature was 75 degrees Fahrenheit. I watched as the red numbers on the thermometer dropped and dropped, until they stopped at 72 degrees. Her foot was actually *colder* than the room! I put her foot up on a stool and covered it with a hot pack; it was half an hour before her leg began to warm even slightly. And when it did heat up, the skin became as red as a lobster. It didn't take a rocket scientist to see that there was something radically wrong with the blood flow in this polio survivor's leg.

Blue Blood and "Polio Feet"

To figure out what was happening, the first thing I did was go back through the medical journals from the polio epidemic years. There actually were a few articles describing changes in blood flow as a result of a poliovirus attack. Two articles from 1951 described exactly what I was seeing in 1982. They said that when polio survivors' limbs cool, skin color changes dramatically, becoming "a blend of violet color varying from reddish violet to a deep dark blue violet." Rehabilitation pioneer Fredrick Kottke said that hours of warming were required to increase skin temperature. He said that polio survivors also felt burning in their cold limbs, which became supersensitive to pain. Kottke and others thought that polio survivors' cold and purple limbs were caused by muscles surrounding the blood vessels going into spasm, narrowing the vessels, reducing the flow of warm blood to the skin, and causing the skin to get very cold. But that explanation didn't make sense to us.

If polio survivors had blood vessel spasms, their legs and feet would be starved for blood and their skin would become white. The blue and violet hues of "polio feet"—a phrase coined by polio survivor and physiatrist Richard Owen—suggested that there was a lot of blood in the legs, or at least lots of deep blue venous blood. And polio survivors having too much blue blood in their veins did make sense. It was known in the 1940s that the poliovirus not only attacked the motor neurons, whose damage and death were responsible for causing paralysis of the muscles that move the limbs, but also attacked and killed sympathetic nervous system neurons inside the spinal cord. It's the sympathetic neurons that make smooth muscle surrounding each blood vessel contract and control how much blood can flow into veins and arteries.

The death of sympathetic neurons should result not in veins and arteries going into spasm, closing down, and stopping blood flow to the skin, but rather in veins being unable to contract and becoming too open, filling with lots of dark blue venous blood.

To find out just what was causing polio feet, we performed our first laboratory study of polio survivors. We placed polio survivors who had one arm more affected by polio than the other and nondisabled subjects in a kind of walk-in refrigerator/oven. We measured both hands' skin temperature, blood flow, how quickly the motor nerves conducted electricity, as well as hand dexterity and strength, at 77 degrees Fahrenheit (25 degrees Celsius), then 86 degrees (30 degrees Celsius) and finally at 68 degrees (20 degrees Celsius).

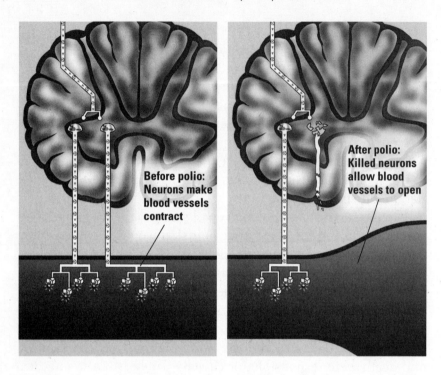

Before polio: Neurons make blood vessels contract

After polio: Killed neurons allow blood vessels to open

CONTROL OF SKIN BLOOD FLOW

What we found explained Margo's experience. Blood flow was significantly lower at 77 degrees in the more affected hand in the post-polio subjects, as compared to their less affected hand or to either hand in nondisabled subjects. Blood flow dropped equally in both hands in both groups as the temperature fell; arteries did not go into spasm and clamp down in the polio survivors as the 1950s researchers had thought. However, as blood flow dropped in polio survivors' more affected hand, so did the ability of its motor nerves to function. At 68 degrees, motor nerve conduction became abnormally slow in 80 percent of polio survivors' more affected hands and in 60 percent of their less affected hands. In fact, motor nerves were functioning as if the room temperature were about 20 degrees *colder* than it actually was. What's more, polio survivors had a 70 percent decrease in manual dexterity and hand strength at 68 degrees, and they told us it took much more effort to move their fingers and lift heavy objects as they got colder.

WHEN THE DEEP PURPLE FALLS

Why do polio survivors lose 70 percent of their strength at a room temperature of 68 degrees Fahrenheit? Why do their nerves function as if they were 20 degrees colder? Why did 60 percent of polio survivors in the 1985 Survey tell us that exposure to cold triggers muscle weakness and pain? The answer is that the size of polio survivors' skin blood vessels can't be regulated because the poliovirus killed off the sympathetic neurons in the spinal cord that are responsible for making the muscles around blood vessels contract.

Here's a typical day in the life of a "blue-blooded" polio survivor:

• You've been in bed all night, toasty warm, with your legs up so that blood is flowing equally to all parts of your body. In the morning your feet are a normal pink color, or maybe even a little red, because your arteries are wide open as a result of the muscles around the arteries being warm and relaxed.

• As your feet go over the side of the bed, gravity pulls blood through those open arteries into the warm and open veins in your legs. As soon as your feet hit the cold tile floor in the bathroom, the heat contained in the warm venous blood near the surface of your skin is transferred to the floor. But your spinal cord can't tell your arteries and veins to contract to limit blood flow and stop the loss of heat.

• As your veins and skin get colder, the arteries also get cold and the muscle around the blood vessels contracts on its own, without the help of sympathetic neurons, decreasing blood flow to the skin and dropping its temperature even farther. Your feet get purple and maybe even dark blue as blood pools in your big, open veins since there isn't enough blood flowing from the arteries to push the blue blood back toward your heart.

- The coldness of your skin moves inside your legs, and the motor nerves—which are just below the surface of the skin—get cold as well. The nerves' ability to conduct signals from your spinal cord to tell your muscles to contract slows, and you start to feel weak.
- The coldness moves more deeply into your legs and chills the muscle, which doesn't contract well when it's cold. The ligaments that connect bone to bone, and tendons that attach muscle to bone, also become cold and less elastic—the same thing that would happen if you put a rubber band in the freezer—and it becomes more difficult for you to move.
- Depending on how much heat you lose, muscles throughout the body will start to contract in preparation for shivering, during which muscles rapidly contract and relax to generate heat. No wonder 30 percent of polio survivors told us in the 2000 Survey that they got extremely cold, sometimes even shivering violently, in the recovery room after having surgery. But even if you don't shiver, and especially if you're sitting in a draft as Margo did, muscle contractions can lead to muscle spasms—especially in the upper back and neck—and trigger muscle and headache pain.

This process of heat loss and deep cooling isn't easy to reverse. Polio survivors report that it may take an hour in a hot bath to warm their thoroughly chilled limbs and allow them to feel less pain and function normally again. But there's also danger in getting too warm. When polio survivors take a long hot bath or spend time in a steaming Jacuzzi, blood vessels do the opposite of what they do in the cold. Polio feet and legs become lobster red as arteries and veins open wide and blood rushes to the skin. When polio survivors stand up, gravity pulls blood into their open vessels and blood pressure can drop, causing light-headedness or possibly even a faint.

Gravity pulling blood into the veins also explains why polio survivors' feet swell when they're hanging down, especially when it's warm. We have found that foot and ankle swelling increase in some polio survivors as they get older, especially in those who have little use of the muscles in their legs, since muscle contractions help pump blood back toward the heart. If your feet are swelling, you need to tell your doctor and make sure that your heart is pumping properly and that your veins and arteries aren't clogged. Our 1985 Survey found that polio survivors don't have more heart trouble than other folk. Our patients don't have more leg blood clots, nor have we seen more than a few polio survivors who have clogged arteries. But anytime you think there's something wrong with your circulation, you should have your heart and blood vessels checked by a doctor who also knows about the cause of "polio feet."

Doctors and polio survivors need to know about the cause of polio feet to prevent the kind of panic that gripped one Nebraska doctor who, upon seeing a blue polio foot, thought that no blood was flowing to the leg and recommended immediate amputation! The patient tried to explain about polio feet, to no avail, but convinced him to call me. I suggested elevating the leg and putting on a hot pack, which produced a warm, red foot that calmed both doctor and patient. As with any other PPS symptom, polio survivors need to be knowledgeable, assert themselves, and advocate for appropriate treatment. Remember: The limb you save will be your own.

Preventing Blue on Blue

What happened to Margo now makes sense. She sat for months in that frigid office, cold air blowing on her shoulders and arms. The ability of her poliovirus-damaged motor neurons to function was being reduced by the cold. She became weaker and more fatigued as her overtaxed, refrigerated motor neurons worked harder day after day to make her cold-stiffened muscles and joints move. Ultimately, enough of those overtaxed neurons failed and probably died under the cold-induced stress to cause permanent weakness in her arms and legs. She became physically and then emotionally blue as she lost both her muscle strength and her ability to work, all for the sake of turning up a thermostat. This shouldn't have happened to Margo and needn't happen to you.

Polio feet and cold intolerance can be easily treated and even prevented. The idea is to stay warm from the get-go. To hold on to your body heat you can get socks, glove liners, clothing—even long johns and leg warmers—made of polypropylene. Sold as Gore-Tex and Thinsulate, polypropylene is a plastic woven into a thin, soft fiber that insulates your skin from the cold but also breathes to prevent you from sweating. Right after getting out of bed or showering, you put on your poly garments and get dressed while your skin is warm and red. To stay warm all day, you can try battery-powered socks or ski-boot heater insoles, which along with poly garments are sold at camping stores and ski shops. It also helps to keep your feet elevated during the day, making it easier for cold blood to flow back to your heart. Dress in layers, too, so that you can control heat loss by changing the amount of clothing covering your body. Whether you're being chilled by a northeast wind in November or by excessive air-conditioning in August, always cover your upper body, especially your neck, to prevent muscle spasms and headaches caused by cold air blowing on your muscles.

It's also helpful to know that polio survivors can have even more trouble when the thermometer goes up and down from day to night and day to day—especially during the transition from summer to fall—than they do once a season settles in. The change of seasons brings increases in symptoms, especially muscle pain and headaches, when polio survivors' temperature-challenged bodies complain as they sweat to lose heat during the day and shiver to conserve heat at night. Layering of clothing is especially important during changes of seasons.

CHILLING EXPERIENCES

There are circumstances when medical personnel need to pay special attention to polio survivors' sensitivity to cold. I've mentioned the higher percentage of polio survivors diagnosed with carpal tunnel syndrome, a compression of the nerves that pass through the wrist into the hand. CTS is diagnosed using a nerve conduction test, the same test we used to learn that polio survivors' nerve conduction slows significantly when they become cold. If polio survivors have a nerve conduction test in a doctor's frigid office, they may be found to have nerve slowing and be diagnosed with CTS, when in reality their nerves are slowed because the room was cold, not because they have nerve compression. Whenever polio survivors have nerve conduction tests, the exam room must be warm for there to be an accurate reading.

Another chilling experience is when polio survivors undergo surgery. In our 2000 Survey 30 percent of polio survivors told us they felt frozen after they had surgery, finding themselves "shaking uncontrollably" in the recovery room, a thoroughly unpleasant and unnecessary situation that a water-filled heating blanket could prevent.

Since we're talking about blood vessels and blood pressure, there are some newly recognized PPS symptoms that are troubling and sometimes dangerous, but can be easily treated with some common sense and a good meal.

CHAPTER 14

Blood Sugar, Blood Pressure, and the Post-Polio Belly

I stood up to begin the meeting and my legs were rubbery. My thoughts became very fuzzy and it was more and more difficult to bring forth the words I wanted to say. I was overwhelmed by fatigue. The frightening thing was that more and more often my brain and body would completely shut down. I could not function until I rested and ate something. But when I ate, the food felt like it got stuck behind my breastbone. Sometimes it took an hour to eat, swallowing small bites, and washing them down with water. Sometimes food won't go down and I have to bring it up. By the time I am done eating I feel a burning in my chest, light-headed, and get overcome by fatigue again. I just have to sleep. When I wake up and I have more energy, I start working. After a while I feel foggy again and need to eat. But then the whole cycle begins anew: The food gets stuck, my stomach gets full, and I have to nap. I never get anything done! My whole life seems to be taken up with eating and sleeping.

TONI, CLASS OF '48

Just when I thought we'd learned everything polio survivors had to teach, something new came up, or to be more precise did not go down.

Toni's description of brain fog isn't unusual for polio survivors. Nor is her swallowing difficulty, which is reported by about 15 percent of Post-Polio Institute patients. But swallowing difficulty is usually mild, with patients reporting that food goes down slowly, or rarely that food or water go "down the wrong pipe," not that food stops moving altogether on its way south. And what about Toni feeling fatigued and needing to eat, but then being so tired after eating she has to go to sleep? If these are PPS symptoms, they're ones we hadn't seen before.

It turns out that these symptoms are PPS. And we already have a basis for understanding their cause and treatment from our discussion of how the poliovirus multiplies in the intestines, how it gets into the brain, and the damage it does to neurons once it gets there.

Into the Bowels of Your Bowels

Back in chapter 3 I tracked the entry of the poliovirus into your body, its multiplying in your intestine, and eventually entering the bloodstream and traveling to your brain. I mentioned that the poliovirus entered your brain and did lots of damage in the brain stem, which contains the reticular formation neurons that not only control brain activation and breathing but also put a brake on how fast your heart beats and how high your blood pressure can go. In addition, other nearby brain stem neurons were damaged by the poliovirus, specifically the neurons that control the vitally important vagus nerve. Vagus neurons also monitor and regulate your blood pressure, and send commands to tell your heart to slow down. The vagus nerve carries commands from brain stem neurons to activate the muscles in your throat, esophagus, stomach, and intestines that make swallowing, digestion, and elimination possible. It also forcefully causes muscles in your stomach to contract, which makes you vomit.

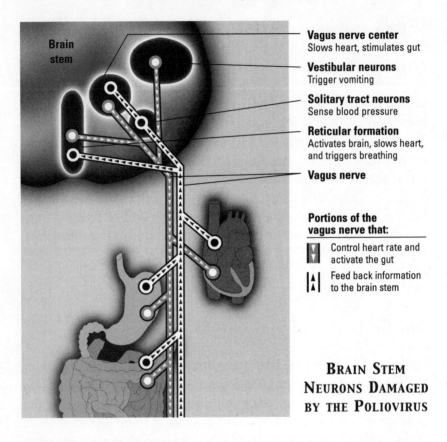

Brain stem

Vagus nerve center
Slows heart, stimulates gut

Vestibular neurons
Trigger vomiting

Solitary tract neurons
Sense blood pressure

Reticular formation
Activates brain, slows heart,
and triggers breathing

Vagus nerve

**Portions of the
vagus nerve that:**

Control heart rate and
activate the gut

Feed back information
to the brain stem

**BRAIN STEM
NEURONS DAMAGED
BY THE POLIOVIRUS**

But the vagus nerve is a two-way street, both sending commands to your heart and gut and listening to the results of those commands. For example, special nerve endings inside your arteries and heart monitor your blood pressure and how hard your heart is beating, sending that information via the vagus nerve to blood pressure control neurons in the brain stem. The vagus also carries information about how much food is inside your throat, esophagus, stomach, and intestines back to those same brain stem neurons.

Given polio survivors' widespread and sometimes severe damage to the brain stem neurons that control heart rate, blood pressure, and the gut, you would expect that there should have been some evidence of this damage back during the poliovirus attack. And there was, especially in those who had the most extensive damage to the brain stem, those diagnosed with "bulbar" polio. Ninety percent of "bulbar" polio patients had obvious damage to the brain stem control center for the vagus nerve. Difficulty swallowing was the most frequent initial bulbar symptom caused by vagus damage. But more dangerous were increased heart rate and blood pressure due to poliovirus damage to other brain stem neurons. Nearly three-quarters of "bulbar" polio patients developed high blood pressure. And although only about 5 percent had uncontrolled increases in heart rate and blood pressure, more than 80 percent of polio patients who experienced this died of cardiovascular collapse.

Past and Present: Hard to Swallow

But, as David Bodian told us, every polio survivor has some degree of "bulbar" polio—some damage to brain stem neurons. So we should expect polio survivors, even those not diagnosed as "bulbar," to have symptoms related to that damage. They did and they do. Right after the poliovirus attack almost 30 percent of patients had nausea and about 50 percent had vomiting and constipation whether or not they had breathing problems, swallowing difficulty, or any muscle paralysis at all. In our 1985 Survey 10 percent of polio survivors reported diarrhea and colitis in midlife, and about 15 percent reported ulcers and constipation, symptoms that are as much as six times more common in polio survivors than in those who've never had polio. These symptoms may be evidence of poliovirus damage to brain stem neurons and the vagus nerve disrupting the normal functioning of the stomach and intestines.

Severe swallowing difficulty is rare among our patients and very few are referred for a video swallow study, which uses a fluoroscope to watch food as it travels over the lips, past the gums, and slides down the esophagus into the stomach. Although swallowing problems are thought to be more common in "bulbar" polio survivors, 60 percent of our patients whose video swallow study revealed that food did not slide right down the esophagus did not have a history of "bulbar" polio. Thus, another Post-Polio Precept:

YOU DON'T HAVE TO HAVE HAD BULBAR POLIO TO HAVE SWALLOWING PROBLEMS TODAY.

Video swallow studies also found that polio survivors have reflux, in which stomach acid moves up into the esophagus and causes heartburn because the muscle controlling the valve between the esophagus and stomach becomes weak. What's more, just as polio survivors' arm and leg muscles get weak, muscles in the throat and esophagus also weaken. We found that muscles in the esophagus can get irritated and go into spasm, just as overworked back and leg muscles do. And that's exactly what we saw in Toni (who didn't have "bulbar" polio) and in other patients reporting pain in their chests when they try to swallow. Toni's video swallow study showed that food stopped moving in her upper esophagus, right at the top of her breastbone, exactly where she reported pain.

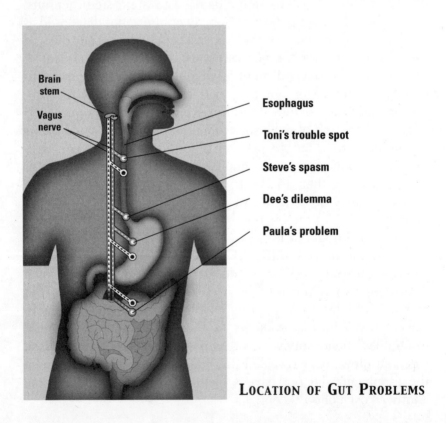

Brain stem

Vagus nerve

Esophagus

Toni's trouble spot

Steve's spasm

Dee's dilemma

Paula's problem

LOCATION OF GUT PROBLEMS

PREVENTING PROBLEMS

Polio survivors who have any swallowing difficulty—especially if they have breathing problems now or had them with their polio attack—need to make sure food and water aren't "going down the wrong pipe," getting into the lungs and potentially causing pneumonia. Although pneumonia is exceedingly rare, please remember this Post-Polio Precept:

IF YOU DEVELOP A NEW BREATHING PROBLEM OR A HINT OF A CHEST INFECTION, SEE A DOCTOR, PRONTO!

Polio survivors need to protect their lungs as they need to protect their neurons.

What's more, doctors themselves need to be vigilant about swallowing difficulties since they may first become evident as a side effect of anesthesia. More than 5 percent of polio survivors in the 2000 Survey reported difficulty swallowing after being given a general anesthetic. But local anesthetics can also cause problems. Since polio survivors are twice as sensitive to pain, they may require more local anesthetic when having dental work. However, the injection of a local anesthetic can result in both pain-conducting nerves and motor nerves being anesthetized. Polio survivors can have trouble if anything further impairs their poliovirus-damaged motor neurons. A local anesthetic can potentially (although rarely) cause tongue and throat muscles to be paralyzed, interfering with swallowing—and possibly breathing—for hours after a tooth is pulled.

TREATING EATING

What's to be done to get food down? Polio survivors with swallowing problems may need a video swallow study to find their cause and make sure something other than PPS isn't causing the trouble. Usually, slowly eating small bites of food, drinking water after each bite, tucking your chin or turning your head to one side when you swallow, swallowing several times, and eating your big meal when you're most rested is all that's needed to treat swallowing problems.

What can Toni and our other "stuck" patients do? We've found that a very low dose of the muscle relaxant clonazapam (Klonopin), taken thirty minutes before eating, relaxes spasms and stops food from sticking in the esophagus. Those who have heartburn, or who think they have ulcers, may have reflux and should talk to their doctors about being evaluated and medications to reduce stomach acid.

Unfortunately, even when Toni was able to swallow with the help of Klonopin we still had to figure out why she was having her most disabling symptoms: feeling tired before she ate and then feeling even more fatigued afterward.

Bottoming Out from the Bottom Up

It turns out that Toni's fatigue after eating was not a new symptom for her. She had always felt tired, sometimes light-headed, and even had to lie down after she'd had a big meal or was constipated and had to strain on the toilet. As she got older, her fatigue after eating and straining had become much worse.

Becoming fatigued when you have a full stomach is not abnormal; it's something that almost everyone experiences after gorging themselves at Thanksgiving. After a big meal, the vagus nerve senses the increased pressure of a full stomach and tells the brain stem neurons, which send out commands to decrease heart rate and increase blood flow to the gut to get nutrients from the food into the blood. This shifting of blood into the belly normally triggers nothing more profound than a small drop in blood pressure and the well-known post-Thanksgiving dinner nap. However, in some polio survivors like Toni, whose vagus nerve and brain stem blood pressure regulation centers are damaged, something much more disabling occurs even after a small meal: Pressure inside the belly, after eating or while straining on the toilet, causes blood pressure to plummet. We monitored Toni's blood pressure and fatigue for weeks and found that it went from 140/85 before eating to 90/55 after even a small meal. The lower her blood pressure, the more fatigued she felt.

Other polio survivors, such as Dee from chapter 10, report that they also have been extremely sensitive to belly pressure and have had lifelong experiences of fainting when they vomited. This makes sense, because vomiting causes tremendous pressure within the belly. But Dee's problem got worse a few years ago when she repeatedly passed out while vomiting. Pressure in her abdomen stimulated the vagus nerve, which actually slowed and then *stopped* her heart for ten seconds at a time, a situation that required her to have a pacemaker implanted.

Some polio survivors, like Linda, report fatigue and light-headedness associated not with heart slowing but heart racing. Like Toni, Linda's symptoms occur when she's eating. But Linda has weakness of the esophagus muscles as well as severe narrowing of its uppermost portion. These problems make swallowing difficult and also cause her heart to race when she tries to force food down. Another polio survivor, Steve, has severe muscle weakness in his esophagus in addition to a muscle spasm of the valve at the bottom of the esophagus, which prevents food from moving into his stomach. When he tries to swallow, food gets stuck just above his stomach and his heart races.

Dropping Like Flies?

The relationships between belly problems, fatigue and fainting, hearts racing and hearts stopping, were very troubling to us, since polio survivors in our 1985 Survey reported belly problems up to six times more frequently than those who hadn't had polio. We were concerned that polio survivors were at higher risk for falling blood pressure, fainting, and even cardiac arrest. So we

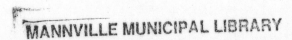

included questions about fainting and fatigue in our 1995 Survey. We found that about half of polio survivors and nondisabled subjects had at least one faint during their lifetimes. The causes of fainting were identical in both groups. So we were relieved that polio survivors were not dropping like flies whenever they had Thanksgiving dinner or got stomach flu. But there was an unexpected finding.

We weren't surprised that three-quarters of the polio survivors, versus only 30 percent of nondisabled participants, rated daily fatigue as moderate or higher. What we didn't anticipate was that both polio survivors and nondisabled subjects who had fainted even *once* during their lifetimes reported significantly higher daily fatigue than those who had never fainted. And polio survivors who had fainted more than three times had the highest fatigue of all. This suggested to us that there is a relationship between fainting and fatigue—that damage to brain stem neurons controlling blood pressure, damage to those controlling heart rate, and damage to the brain-activation neurons is related in anyone who has chronic fatigue, whether they've had polio or not.

This notion is interesting because it links fatigue in polio survivors to fatigue in those who have chronic fatigue syndrome. In 1995 pediatrician Peter Rowe found that some patients with CFS have fatigue that is associated with a drop in blood pressure when they stand up. Fatigue also increased in some CFS patients when they take a hot shower or are in a hot room. Rowe's observations paralleled the finding from our 1985 Survey that fatigue increased in more than one-third of polio survivors when they were exposed to heat. Another parallel with polio survivors was Rowe's observation that a CFS patient had "a purple discoloration" of her feet and hands after standing. This discoloration was reported in patients with chronic fatigue back in 1959 and is remarkably similar to the color of "polio feet."

These findings indicate that some CFS patients have lost the ability to regulate the size of their veins, just like polio survivors, allowing blood to pool and blood pressure to drop. Chronic fatigue related to blood pooling in veins that are too open is seen in another condition called POTS (postural orthostatic tachycardia syndrome). This is associated with an increase in heart rate when patients stand up, as well as with several other now-familiar symptoms: light-headedness, constipation, slowing of the intestines, or bloating after eating. Nearly 50 percent of POTS patients report that symptoms began after a viral illness. So polio survivors, patients with CFS, and POTS share fatigue plus abnormalities of blood vessels and bellies, blood pressure and heart rate, that seem to be related to brain stem neurons not functioning normally, probably as a result of damage by a virus.

What's to be done about bottoming out? Polio survivors and anyone with chronic fatigue should have their heart rate and blood pressure taken while lying, sitting, and, if possible, standing. If fatigue is associated with either a heart rate increase or a drop in blood pressure, compression stockings are often helpful to stop blood from pooling in the legs. You can also go to a *low* blood pressure specialist and ask about medications that increase the amount of fluid in your blood or reduce the size of your veins to stop blood from pooling.

Gut-Wrenching Experiences

Here's a song we've heard before, but with an added verse—neck pain and headache:

> When I am overly tired my heart starts pounding, and then it seems to stop for a second or two—not just a skipped beat, but a complete stop! I get a sick headache with neck pain. I feel nauseated, diarrhea is imminent, and I feel as though I will faint. I feel trembly and weak in my muscles. I lie on the couch for nearly an hour and things begin to calm down, though I am left feeling pretty zapped.
>
> PAULA, CLASS OF '43

Paula's description sounds very much like polio survivor William O. Douglas's report: "Concentrated exercise . . . made me feel faint; and sometimes I'd be sick at my stomach or get a severe headache." Patients tell me they have "migraine" headaches because they have pain on one side of their head that is associated with nausea. Despite the nausea, most polio survivors don't have migraines. What happens is that the muscles on one side of the neck go into spasm, causing neck pain and a one-sided headache. The spasm pushes on the vagus nerve, slows the heart, drops the blood pressure, and turns on the gut, causing nausea and maybe a feeling of faintness—all because the functioning of the vagus nerve is discombobulated.

What makes this worse is that polio survivors seem to have a penchant for nausea and vomiting, which can first reveal itself when they are given anesthetics. There's no question that the ether given when polio survivors had childhood surgeries caused severe nausea and vomiting. But even today's modern anesthetics can cause severe and prolonged vomiting in survivors, probably because of poliovirus damage to the vestibular neurons, the brain's vomiting center. In the 2000 Survey just over 20 percent of polio survivors told us they vomited anywhere from several hours to several days after having surgery. Especially since polio survivors may be more apt to faint when they throw up, it's essential that antivomiting medication be given both before and after surgery. This medication is also indispensable for polio survivors receiving radiation and chemotherapy.

Another cause of vomiting after surgery is intestinal paralysis, where the intestine just stops moving and the food has nowhere to go but back from whence it came. Some of our patients have developed paralyzed intestines not only after abdominal surgery, when drugs are intentionally given to slow the activity of the vagus nerve, but also for no apparent reason at all. Polio survivors need to be careful whenever they are given drugs that are anticholinergic—drugs that block the action of acetylcholine, the neurochemical released by the vagus nerve that activates the muscles of the intestine.

Finding relationships between fatigue, swallowing difficulties, low blood pressure, and the abnormal functioning of poliovirus-damaged brain stem neurons still does not explain Toni's very first symptom, the severe brain fog when she hasn't eaten.

Blood Sugar and the Post-Polio Neuron

You may have heard that science is 1 percent inspiration and 99 percent perspiration. As you've seen with our "discoveries" about polio survivors—their Type A behavior, sensitivity to cold, and twitching at night—science can also be 99 percent observation, just plain old listening to your patients. But sometimes you discover something through circumstances you would never have anticipated. That's what happened with our discovery of polio survivors' problems with blood sugar.

Susan Creange, a doctoral candidate and intern at The Post-Polio Institute, was looking for a dissertation topic. Since she was interested in hypoglycemia, low blood sugar, I suggested she investigate whether there was a relationship between blood sugar, fatigue, and attention problems in polio survivors. Susan discovered more than we ever imagined.

Susan recruited polio survivors with varying levels of fatigue and carefully screened out those with any medical condition that could cause fatigue, including sleep disorders, a slow thyroid, and diabetes. She asked what subjects ate during a typical day and found that many polio survivors eat a "Type A diet": They drink several cups of coffee for breakfast, skip lunch, and eat pizza for dinner before going out in the evening to their second job.

Susan then measured polio survivors' blood sugar and gave them the same tests of attention and memory that we'd used since 1992 to study polio survivors with fatigue. She found that the lower polio survivors' blood sugar, the worse they did on the most difficult attention tests. Attention was about 20 percent below normal for those whose blood sugars were around eighty, which is at the bottom of the normal range for blood sugar. In fact, polio survivors' ability to pay attention with a blood sugar of eighty was actually worse than in diabetics with a blood sugar of sixty-five! In terms of focusing attention, then, polio survivors' brains act as if they were hypoglycemic, blood sugar levels about fifteen points lower than the actual measurement. This finding illustrates another Post-Polio Precept:

A BORDERLINE LOW RESULT ON A BLOOD TEST SHOULD BE CONSIDERED ABNORMAL IN A POLIO SURVIVOR.

Fatigued polio survivors with borderline low anemia or thyroid functioning should be treated, even though other patients would not. Given their difficulties with the brain-activating system, polio survivors don't have a "safety zone" as do those who didn't have polio.

HYPOGLYCEMIA: MORE REAL THAN APPARENT

Why would the brain-activating neurons in polio survivors with normal blood sugar levels function as if there were too little sugar in the blood? We already have enough information about poliovirus damage to the brain to understand what may be happening.

Just as with the poliovirus, receptors grab on to molecules of sugar in the intestine, move it into the blood, which carries it to the brain. Brain blood vessels also have blood sugar receptors that grab on to sugar molecules and pull them into the brain. Sugar is the only fuel neurons can use. The brain, which is only about 2 percent of your body weight, uses half of all the sugar in your blood. And the more challenging the mental task—like those difficult attention tests—the more sugar neurons need to function. But for sugar to get inside the neurons, yet another group of receptors on the surface of the neurons must latch on to the sugar molecules to pull them inside. And that's where the problems likely begin.

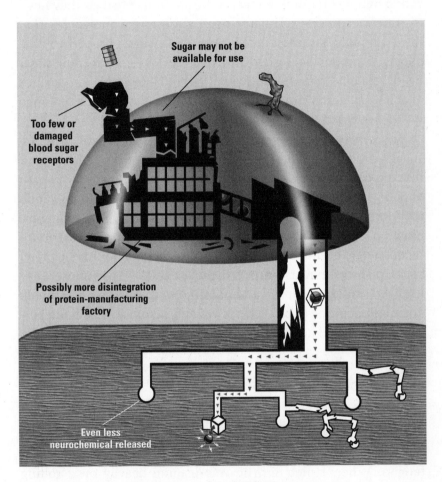

Too few or
damaged
blood sugar
receptors

Sugar may not be
available for use

Possibly more disintegration
of protein-manufacturing
factory

Even less
neurochemical released

Hypoglycemic PPS Neuron

Just like the poliovirus receptor, sugar receptors are made of protein. You know that the protein factories inside motor neurons are breaking apart in polio survivors experiencing new muscle weakness, and that there is a partial plugging of neurons' tubules—the microscopic pipes that carry protein and nutrients throughout the neuron. If there is similar damage inside brain-activating system neurons, polio survivors may not make enough protein to manufacture all the sugar receptors that brain-activating neurons require to take in the amounts of sugar they need to function properly. What's more, the protein molecules that make up blood sugar receptors may not be made properly by the damaged protein factories, and may be less able to pull sugar inside. Finally, if the tubules are clogged, large enough quantities of sugary fuel may not be able to get where they need to go once inside brain-activating neurons.

There may also be a double whammy with regard to blood sugar, as there has been with other aspects of PPS. Motor neurons' protein factories are seen to break apart, not only as a result of poliovirus infection, but also in animals that are starving. Polio survivors' neurons may always be partially starved due to a combination of overuse and an inability to take in and distribute blood sugar. An unsatisfied demand for large amounts of blood sugar, due to survivors' Type A lifestyles and overuse-abuse, may itself be starving neurons and causing protein factories to break apart and neurons to fail. This is yet another reason for polio survivors to follow The Golden Rule.

ARE ALL SYMPTOMS PPS?

Bill looked like a severe, but not unusual, PPS patient. He came to us complaining of muscle weakness and overwhelming fatigue. When I met him he was leaning heavily on a rolling walker and could hardly stay awake. His head resting in his hands, he couldn't remember the questions I was asking, let alone give me answers. A clear case of post-polio muscle weakness, and brain fatigue, yes? Well, no.

We measured Bill's blood sugar—and found that it was 350! I called his doctor, who gave him oral medication for diabetes, and his sugar came down to a normal 105. As Bill's blood sugar decreased, so did his muscle weakness and fatigue. He "woke up," grew mentally sharp, and discarded the walker.

Bill's story again underscores that all PPS are diagnosed by exclusion. It is crucial that all potential causes for new symptoms be ruled out before a diagnosis of PPS is made. Bill's PPS symptoms were in fact the result of his diabetes and very high blood sugar having a terrible effect on his poliovirus-damaged spinal cord and brain-activating system neurons. Once medication treated his diabetes, his post-polio neurons could eat hearty and function well again.

You should also know that there is a medication that actually prevents neurons from eating well. Steroids, such as prednisone, are the most powerful of anti-inflammatory medications; they're sometimes given when polio survivors have serious lung infections. But being anti-inflammatory, steroids are sometimes given when doctors can't figure out what else to do for polio survivors' joint pain when nonsteroidal anti-inflammatory drugs, like ibuprofen, don't help. Unfortunately, steroids block neurons' ability to take in blood sugar—not exactly helpful when polio survivors have trouble taking in blood sugar all by themselves. So here's another Post-Polio Precept:

POLIO SURVIVORS SHOULD NOT TAKE STEROIDS UNLESS THEY HAVE A SERIOUS MEDICAL CONDITION, AND THEY SHOULD NOT TAKE STEROIDS FOR PAIN.

Serious medical conditions would include pneumonia, asthma, and rheumatoid arthritis. But as you know from chapter 10, the treatment of osteoarthritis and joint pain—for all PPS—is neither a steroid nor any other medication but taking the load off overused limbs and following The Golden Rule.

BLOOD SUGAR AND EMOTIONAL STRESS

The likelihood of a shortage of blood sugar receptors on poliovirus-damaged neurons in the brain-activating system and spinal cord may help explain the unexpected finding in our 1985 Survey that emotional stress was reported to be the second most common trigger for PPS symptoms. In chapter 9 I mentioned that cortisol, the body's internally manufactured steroid and its main antistress hormone, may be the missing link between emotional stress and muscle weakness, because cortisol interferes with neurons' ability to sprout, to make proteins, and to use blood sugar. Having too few blood sugar receptors on poliovirus-damaged neurons may conspire with cortisol to starve spinal cord motor neurons when they most need sugar—when you're under stress—and cause stress-induced muscle weakness.

Polio survivors' fatigue during stress may also be caused by the combination of too much cortisol and too few blood sugar receptors. The stressful attention tests we give to polio survivors cause even nondisabled folk to report fatigue, decreased energy, trouble focusing attention, and drowsiness, symptoms that are found to increase as their bodies produce more cortisol. What's more, cortisol not only prevents neurons from taking up blood sugar and inhibits the manufacture of proteins, but also directly slows the activity of reticular formation neurons. Even worse, people who are Type A release more cortisol in response to stress, and it takes longer for cortisol to return to normal levels. Finally, a shortage of blood sugar receptors in the poliovirus-damaged hypothalamus may prevent it from "knowing" when sugar is low and stop it from releasing the brain activating hormone ACTH. This may explain our finding that fatigued polio survivors do not release ACTH in response to stress, and that the more fatigue polio survivors report, the less ACTH they release. Is it any wonder that emotional stress plays havoc with polio survivors' bodies and brains?

THE PROOF OF THE STUDIES IS IN THE EATING

What does all of this sweet talk tell us about treating PPS? It suggests that polio survivors should eat the way hypoglycemic people do. So we did a study, placing Toni and other patients who reported increased symptoms as they got farther from a meal on a hypoglycemia diet. They decreased the amount of carbohydrates they ate—bread, starchy vegetables, and sweets—and increased their protein intake, since protein provides a long-lasting, slow-release source of blood sugar. Patients increased protein at each meal and added a small snack containing protein in the morning and afternoon. They rated their symptoms before and after starting the diet. It wasn't more than a day or so before their brain fog lifted. Overall, patients reported an 80 percent decrease in both fatigue and difficulty focusing attention on the hypoglycemia diet.

To see if polio survivors in general report a relationship between what they eat—or *don't* eat—and PPS symptoms, we asked polio survivors to list what they usually ate for breakfast and rate their symptoms as part of our 1998 International Survey of 350 polio survivors and people without disabilities. We found that the typical post-survivor's breakfast consisted of coffee, a slice of toast, and sometimes cold cereal, which provided about nine grams of protein. The polio survivors weighed 160 pounds on average, which means that their bodies needed to take in seventy-four grams of protein each day to maintain their weight. If you split that seventy-four grams into four parts—breakfast, lunch, dinner, and the combined morning and afternoon snacks—polio survivors should have been eating eighteen grams of protein at breakfast, not nine. The farther polio survivors got from the eighteen grams of protein they should have been eating at breakfast, the more fatigue, muscle weakness, and pain they reported during the day. And the more protein they were missing at breakfast, the more cups of caffeine-loaded coffee or tea they were drinking, probably to wake up their sugar-starved brains.

THE POST-POLIO PROTEIN "DIET"

What should polio survivors do to treat their hidden hypoglycemia? They need to eat three to five times a day and have protein at each meal, especially at breakfast. We recommend that polio survivors eat immediately after they get up, since they need to break their fast and "fill their gas tanks" for the day ahead before stressing hungry neurons by bathing and dressing.

The number of grams of protein you need to eat during the day is based on your body weight:

Grams of Protein Each Day = Pounds of Body Weight x 0.46

If you want to maintain a weight of 160 pounds, you should eat seventy-four grams of protein. Divide this number by four—breakfast, lunch, dinner, and the two snacks—and you should be eating about eighteen grams of protein at each meal and nine grams for each snack.

Here are some good and not-so-good breakfast and snack ideas. Look for low-calorie foods that have more grams of protein than they do fat. Pick an array of different breakfasts and snacks so you can have variety throughout the day and the week:

	Protein (grams)	Fat (grams)
GREAT:		
Cottage cheese (lite, 1 cup)	28	2
Salmon (3 ounces)	17	5
Yogurt (8 ounces)	12	4
Tofu (6 ounces)	10	6
Milk (8 ounces or 1 cup)		
Skim-plus milk	11	0
2% milk	8	3
Soy milk	7	5
2 egg whites	7	0
Bagel (Lenders)	6	1
Egg Beaters (1/4 cup)	5	0

	Protein (grams)	Fat (grams)
SNACK BARS:		
MET-Rx		
Fudge Brownie	26	3
Source One	15	3
GeniSoy Bar	14	4
Balance Bar	14	6
Cliff (Luna) Bar	10	5
PROTEIN DRINKS:		
MET-Rx powder in 2% milk	46	6
Designer Protein Powder in 2% milk	26	3
Carnation Instant Breakfast in 2% milk	12	3
HIGHER FAT:		
Swiss cheese (1 ounce)	8	8
Lite n' Lively cheese (1 ounce)	6	4
Hard-boiled egg	6	6
Peanut butter (1 tablespoon)	4	4
Cream cheese (lite, 1 ounce)	3	5
LOWER PROTEIN:		
Quaker Life cereal (1 ounce)	5	2
English muffin	5	1
Oatmeal (1 package)	4	2
Cheerios (1 ounce)	4	2
Shredded Wheat (1 ounce)	3	1
Total cereal (1 cup)	3	1

	Protein (grams)	Fat (grams)
NOT GOOD:		
Egg McMuffin	17	32
Bacon (3 strips)	6	10
Coffee	0	0

Although this "diet" is focused on protein as a long-lasting source of blood sugar, we aren't recommending an all-protein, no-carbohydrate diet to lose weight. We aren't recommending a diet at all, but for you to take in the amount of protein your neurons need. As for carbohydrates, we tell our patients that a portion of bread or potatoes should be the same as a portion of meat: about the size of a deck of playing cards. You also need to eat a selection of fruits and low-starch vegetables each day.

A RED HERRING

No, not a herring you eat; a herring that doctors who know nothing about PPS try to feed you. Many polio survivors have been told by doctors that if they'd only lose twenty or ten or even five pounds, their PPS symptoms would disappear. Weight loss curing PPS is the red herring.

Post-polio researcher Margaret Campbell found that weight was not related to any PPS symptom. A four-year study of U.S. and Swedish polio survivors found that American polio survivors were ten pounds heavier to begin with and gained eight pounds over four years, compared to the Swedes gaining one and a half pounds. Still, Americans had no greater loss in strength or increase in any PPS symptoms than did the lighter Swedes. Sure, if you're five foot one and weigh in at 250, you need to drop some pounds. But losing weight is not the cure for PPS.

Our patients also worry that stopping exercise, resting more, and eating more protein will cause them to gain weight. One of our patients proved the opposite. Abby, a programming whiz at AT&T, charted on his computer the number of grams of protein he ate and how many steps he took during the day; he weighed himself once a week. We had given him braces and crutches plus a scooter, and told him to rest. He religiously ate protein at breakfast and for snacks, limited portion sizes, and reduced fats. Abby lost a pound and a half each week. Other patients have had similar results, or have found that their weight did not increase when they slowed down and even sat down.

And if you want to lose weight, you can enter your target weight into the formula to calculate the amount of protein you should be eating. For example, if you weigh 160 and want to weigh 145, you should eat sixty-seven grams of protein each day. But please check with your doctor and have your cholesterol, thyroid, and blood sugar measured before changing your eating habits and trying to lose weight.

PART THREE

A New Beginning

CHAPTER 15

Mind Over Matter

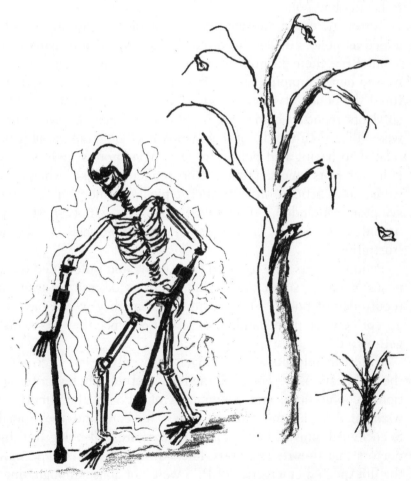

ALICE RUMPLER, CLASS OF '22

If a picture is worth a thousand words, then this drawing by artist and polio survivor Alice Rumpler is worth an entire chapter on the psychology of PPS. This image makes visible polio survivors' terror when the buried skeleton of polio returns, walking on new forearm crutches, bringing with it polio's past and ushering in its sequel. Ninety percent of polio survivors in the 1985 Survey reported that they never even considered the possibility of developing new problems after having reached maximum recovery from polio. Nearly three-quarters did not initially think that their new symptoms were in any way related to having had polio.

Terror increased and confusion, frustration, and anger were added as polio survivors were confronted by doctors' ignorance about PPS, their disinterest and disdain. Many physicians dismissed new symptoms as "psychosomatic" or as being "manufactured" by polio survivors. In our 1985 Survey a quarter of polio survivors reported being told by physicians that the symptoms were "all in their minds" or that symptoms "could not possibly be related to having had polio." In Mary Westbrook's 1991 survey polio survivors reported that doctors replied "rubbish" when they were shown articles on PPS; their typical comments about new symptoms included, "It was just nerves . . . empty nest syndrome . . . boredom . . . laziness . . . hypochondriasis . . . sexual frustration."

Polio survivors also received frightening and unfounded diagnoses, such as "some kind of Lou Gehrig's disease" or even "a recurrence of polio." Many were told that they would have to accept new symptoms and loss of function since they were "just getting old."

Unfortunately, little has changed in twenty years. Even after the publication of scores of medical journal articles, international conferences, and acceptance of PPS by the American Medical Association—and even by Medicare and the Social Security Administration—polio survivors are still being told by doctors that they're lazy, crazy, fat, old, or just plain lying. As if the unexpected emergence of PPS were not abuse enough, doctors continue to thoughtlessly and needlessly add new chapters to the volumes of emotional abuse polio survivors have already experienced.

The Double Whammy

The occurrence of PPS itself provides a double emotional slap in the face. Not only do polio survivors have to deal with the emotions surrounding PPS symptoms and the limitations they bring, but also they are being outed by those symptoms and limitations. One-quarter of polio survivors in our 1985 Survey, regardless of their physical limitations, told us that they did not think of themselves as having any disability before developing PPS. With the onset of PPS, nearly half admitted to having two disabilities: polio and PPS. So survivors must face the emotional reality of PPS as they are simultaneously forced to confront the long-buried, deeply hidden, or never addressed feelings associated with polio itself.

And feelings associated with polio were often deeply buried under years of hospitalization, physical therapy, multiple surgeries, impressive accomplishments, and denial by polio survivors of their own fundamental physical and emotional needs. It's not surprising that some of our patients have never spoken the word *polio*, have never told even their spouses that they'd been touched by The Dread Disease. Nor is it surprising that our 1995 Survey found that polio survivors who were hospitalized for long periods, those who were not treated with concern by medical staff, and those who were abused are today the most sensitive to criticism, are the most Type A, and are having the greatest difficulty dealing psychologically with PPS.

And of course, there is the most painful Polio Paradox of all:

TYPE A BEHAVIOR THAT WAS SO WELL TAUGHT AND SO WELL LEARNED—THE VERY WAY OF LIFE THAT POLIO SURVIVORS BELIEVED ALLOWED THEM TO ESCAPE "MORTAL DANGER," APPEAR "NORMAL," AND REENTER SOCIETY—IS ITSELF THE CAUSE OF OVERUSE-ABUSE THAT HAS BEATEN UP POLIO-DAMAGED BODIES AND TRIGGERED PPS.

Becoming normal has taken a heavy toll. Polio survivors lived by the "Good Chart" and their neurons are dying by the "Good Chart."

The Great Depression

Let's say this right up front: If you weren't depressed about having PPS or losing hard-won functional abilities, you *would* be crazy. Imagine someone *liking* being told that they needed to wear a brace, use crutches, or get a wheelchair.

But there's depressed and there's *depressed*. In the 1990 Survey just over half of polio survivors told us that they felt "sad," and nearly a quarter said they had at some point been diagnosed with depression. Clinical depression, what's called a "major depressive episode," isn't just feeling sad. To be diagnosed with clinical depression, you would be sad, but you'd also have other symptoms: decreased enjoyment of life, an inability to sleep or sleeping too much, decreased activity during the day, fatigue or loss of energy, an inability to think or concentrate, decreased appetite, thoughts of suicide, and feelings of worthlessness or guilt. I'm sure you noticed that all of these symptoms—except decreased appetite, thoughts of suicide, and maybe worthlessness—are commonly reported by those with PPS. More than 60 percent of Post-Polio Institute patients report that they don't enjoy life the way they used to; about half say they're sad, anxious, critical of and disappointed in themselves; just over a third say they have decreased interest in other people and cry frequently; and about a quarter report decreased appetite or increased guilt. Despite these symptoms being common in our patients, only about 15 percent actually meet the diagnostic criteria for a major depressive episode. Still, that's at least twice the rate of depression in the general population.

What's more interesting than the frequency of depression in our patients is that depression and even sadness are not related to post-polio symptoms themselves. Polio survivors don't report that they are sad, let alone depressed, when they develop fatigue, muscle weakness, or pain, even if those symptoms are severe. Sadness and depression—decreased enjoyment, poor appetite, and increased guilt—appear in our patients when PPS symptoms interfere with their ability to work, meet social obligations, and care for themselves or their homes. Polio survivors get depressed when they can no longer meet other people's expectations and do what they think they "should." It won't be a surprise to you that the patients who are the most sad, guilty, and tearful are the most sensitive to criticism by others and are most likely to think of themselves as failures.

Treating Depression

If you are thought to be depressed, it's essential that your doctor understand the overlap between symptoms of depression and PPS, and that treatable causes for depressive symptoms be ruled out, such as having a slow thyroid, anemia, or a sleep disorder. These conditions should be treated before an antidepressant is prescribed.

And what about antidepressants? Very few of our patients who have a clinical depression are given an antidepressant. We treat depression in psychotherapy, where the overwhelming majority of patients get better quickly without medication. But except for the potential for some antidepressants to cause daytime sleepiness, there is no reason that a polio survivor shouldn't take an antidepressant if one is needed. The SSRIs (selective serotonin reuptake inhibitors) such as Prozac, Paxil, Zoloft, and Celexa are effective and have fewer side effects than the older tricyclic antidepressants, such as Elavil (amitriptyline), which make you sleepy, cause dry mouth and constipation, and can make your blood pressure drop when you stand up. SSRIs are somewhat stimulating and can cause insomnia, nausea, and decreased sexual interest or ability. The even newer non-SSRI antidepressants are also effective and sometimes have fewer side effects. Wellbutrin is more stimulating and has fewer sexual side

effects than SSRIs. As we discussed, Remeron, Serzone, and trazodone are so sedating that each can be used as a sleeping pill in
those very few instances when polio survivors should use
sleeping pills, such as when they are getting used to a PAP
machine.

Regardless of the method—psychotherapy alone or therapy
plus medication—treating depression is doubly important in
polio survivors, not only because depression should always be
treated but also because depression is a major cause of patients
refusing treatment for PPS. We found that just over 60 percent
of patients who refused treatment for PPS and 50 percent of
those who left treatment were clinically depressed. If a polio survivor is too depressed to begin or continue with treatment,
therapy and even an antidepressant should be started right away
(keep in mind that it can take up to five weeks for the medication to kick in and help you feel better).

Less Isn't Always More

Alice's drawing illustrates the fear, depression, and hopelessness
that can arise with PPS. These powerful emotions combine with
a denial of new symptoms and sensitivity to criticism to create
the most important and difficult Polio Paradox regarding managing PPS:

**THE TYPE A BEHAVIOR THAT SUPPOSEDLY PROTECTED
AGAINST CRITICISM AND FEELINGS OF FAILURE IS
PREVENTING POLIO SURVIVORS FROM CARING FOR
THEMSELVES AND MANAGING THEIR PPS.**

Over the past twenty years, 16 percent of polio survivors who
came to us for evaluation refused any treatment for PPS, while
12 percent who began therapy left treatment because they were
not able to make the changes necessary to manage their PPS.
Unfortunately, rejecting change is the rule among polio survivors. A post-polio clinic in Michigan reported that more than

40 percent of patients who had been prescribed a brace used it only "sporadically" and that 70 percent refused to use a new cane or crutch simply because they "didn't want to." Doctors at a Wisconsin post-polio clinic concluded that the major reason for failure of PPS symptoms to improve was "the unwillingness of the patient to follow any of the recommendations made."

In chapter 9 we discussed physiatrist Paul Peach following the progress of his post-polio patients, over several years. He found that just over one-third followed all the treatment recommendations, over one-third made some changes, but 20 percent did nothing he suggested. Just over 30 percent refused braces and nearly 50 percent refused lifestyle changes. The same thing happens at The Post-Polio Institute, where about one-third of patients adopt a "Chinese menu" approach to managing PPS—picking a disabled parking sticker and a brace from "Column A" but refusing the cane or to take breaks at work in "Column B." Patients who pick and choose—those who only partially care for themselves—report that symptoms continue to increase one month after graduating from The Post-Polio Institute program. Those who fully care for themselves by adopting all of our recommendations have reductions in symptoms and increases in well-being:

Change in Symptoms One Month after Graduation from the Post-Polio Institute Program

	Partial Self-Care	Full Self-Care
Difficulty with:		
Concentrating	35%	-20%
Household activities	25%	-5%
Memory	15%	-5%
Staying awake	15%	-20%
Walking outside	13%	-5%
Weakness	10%	-10%
Sitting up in bed	10%	-25%
Getting out of a chair	5%	-15%

	Partial Self-Care	Full Self-Care
Thinking	5%	-30%
Feeling tired	15%	-30%
Muscle weakness	10%	-11%
Worrying about health	10%	-30%
Expecting to get better	0%	20%
Interest in sex	-15%	50%
Feeling:		
Like a failure	10%	-70%
Satisfaction in life	-25%	30%

Certainly, doing something to help yourself is better than doing nothing. But these changes in symptoms make clear that polio survivors can't afford to pick and choose what they're going to do to manage PPS.

Does following the "Chinese menu" approach have a long term effect on PPS symptoms? Remember that Paul Peach found polio survivors who followed only some of his treatment recommendations lost about 3 percent of their muscle strength per year, while those who did everything they needed to do actually gained just over 1 percent per year. We found the same kind of changes in our patients' symptoms at their re-evaluation one year after graduation:

Change in Symptoms One Year after Graduation
from the Post-Polio Institute Program

	Partial Self-Care	Full Self-Care
Difficulty with:		
Social Activities	51%	-47%
Getting out of a chair	45%	-29%
Household activities	41%	-15%
Self-Care	36%	-16%
Working	34%	-42%

	Partial Self-Care	Full Self-Care
Sitting up in bed	29%	-29%
Thinking	23%	-40%
Memory	16%	-10%
Sleeping	13%	-29%
Mind wandering	13%	-13%
Attention	2%	-33%
Concentrating	0%	-36%
Walking inside	0%	-19%
Pain interferes with activities	0%	-24%
Feeling:		
Like a failure	54%	-73%
Tired	22%	-43%
Sad	20%	-57%
Satisfaction in life	-38%	43%

These findings reinforce that polio survivors must do everything that can help to decrease their symptoms if they are going to get better and stay better, and underscore this fundamental Post-Polio Precept:

THE ONLY CAUSE OF PROGRESSION OF MUSCLE WEAKNESS IS POLIO SURVIVORS NOT TAKING CARE OF THEMSELVES.

Of course the big question is *why* many polio survivors don't do all they can to feel better.

COMING AND GOING

Although we began to ask back in 1985, why polio survivors have such trouble taking care of themselves, we didn't have a complete answer until we combined the findings of the 1985, 1990, and 1995 Post-Polio Surveys. It turns out that there's a chain of events that began way back when you had polio that determines whether or not you'll even come in to have your PPS symptoms evaluated:

- If you had polio later in the century and were young when you had polio, you are more likely to have been abused and are more sensitive to criticism and failure . . .
- If you are more sensitive to criticism and failure, were not treated with concern by medical staff when you had polio, and were hospitalized for surgeries or rehabilitation, you are more Type A today . . .
- If you are more Type A today and if your questions of medical personnel were not answered at all when you had polio, you won't come in for evaluation.

When polio survivors do come in for evaluation, which ones refuse treatment? In the 1995 Survey we found that men are less likely to agree to treatment, as are those who are clinically depressed, those who are more Type A, and those who did not have their questions answered with concern by medical staff back when they had polio.

And once polio survivors begin treatment, which will drop out? They're older, half are clinically depressed, and they're 30 percent more Type A and just over 20 percent more sensitive to criticism and failure than patients who stay.

Finally, when polio survivors come for evaluation and stick with treatment, which follow the Chinese menu approach and which take the full self-care route? The partial self-care patients are the usual suspects: They're older, more sensitive to criticism and failure, and more Type A. Our 1997 study found that the more Type A patients are, the less likely it is they'll take two fifteen-minute breaks each day.

Truth be told, we don't expect our patients to do everything they need to do to manage their PPS every minute of every day. The fundamental goal of The Post-Polio Institute program is simply to help polio survivors turn off their Type A autopilot and start making their *own* decisions about what they're going to do—and not do—to manage PPS and preserve their remaining, poliovirus-damaged neurons. But to do this, polio survivors need a little help from their friends.

All in the Family

Given polio survivors' painful history of mistreatment by society and sometimes by their own parents, acceptance by others—especially by their families—would be expected to have a profound effect on their willingness to come out of the closet and manage their PPS. Our 1994 study found that polio survivors who complete treatment say that their families "would always help me in any kind of trouble." Margaret Campbell found that family support increases acceptance of PPS in polio survivors who have new physical limitations, and both Campbell and psychologist Denise Tate both found more symptoms of depression in polio survivors who have less social and family support.

But polio survivors' fear of rejection by those closest to them is nowhere more evident than in the findings of Mary Westbrook. She discovered that the lifestyle changes most obvious to family members—asking family for help, buying special equipment, and making home modifications—were adopted by the fewest polio survivors despite their rating these changes as the most effective in helping manage PPS. Swedish researcher Anna-Lisa Thoren-Jonsson found that more than 50 percent of polio survivors depend on others for cleaning, shopping, and transportation. Yet these same polio survivors rejected about half of the special equipment recommended to help them. It's no surprise that our 1997 study, which included a questionnaire measuring how polio survivors felt about themselves, found that patients who use crutches or a wheelchair felt less adequate as family members.

So it's essential that family members actively support lifestyle changes and understand polio survivors' need to feel valuable despite their reduced physical activity and appearing "more disabled" as the result of using necessary assistive devices. This is why, after four weeks of treatment at The Post-Polio Institute, the entire treatment team meets with patients, their families, and sometimes even their friends, coworkers, and employers. Since patients and family have already read *The Post-Polio Workbook* and watched our videotape about the cause and treatment of PPS, we answer any questions about PPS, explain the reasons we're recommending specific assistive devices and changes in lifestyle, and help divvy up the chores—shopping, cooking, cleaning, laundry—among family members. It's rare that family members don't come to the meeting (when patients are willing to ask them to come), and rarer still that family and friends don't readily agree to take some of the physical load off patients. Husbands are often eager to do shopping, cleaning, and laundry, saying about their wives, "I've been asking her to let me help for years. She just won't stop!" Still, most polio survivors feel that they are a burden to their families when they ask for help. The true burden for families is seeing loved ones in pain and unable to function, not being asked to take out the garbage. In twenty years we have never had a "post-polio divorce."

Many polio survivors feel they are burdening their families, not only by asking for physical help but also by talking about how they feel. So many polio survivors have told me, "I don't want to trouble other people with my feelings." But since feelings have a way of making themselves known whether you want them to or not, and even whether you're aware of them or not, let me give you another Post-Polio Precept:

IRRITABILITY IS NOT A REAL EMOTION.

If you are irritable as a bear, if you start sniping at your spouse, yelling at traffic, or kicking the cat, there is a real emotion inside of you that's trying to get out. Better to tell your spouse what you feel—or even that you're irritable and don't know what you feel—than to pick a fight. Since Margaret Campbell found that family communication and support significantly reduce polio survivors' symptoms of depression and emotional stress, talking about feelings will not only help you and your family feel better emotionally, but also will decrease your stress-triggered symptoms.

DRAG AND DROP

Since family support is usually so helpful, I was surprised years ago to find that there is such a thing as families being *too* helpful and to discover this Polio Paradox:

PATIENTS ACCOMPANIED TO THE PPS EVALUATION BY A SPOUSE, FRIEND, OR FAMILY MEMBER WERE LESS LIKELY TO COMPLETE TREATMENT.

If family support is so helpful, this paradox makes no sense. But it's actually a variation on the old saw, "You can lead a horse to water but you can't make him drink." You can drag polio survivors to The Post-Polio Institute but you can't make them change, physically or emotionally, or stop them from dropping out of treatment.

We have seen a similar phenomenon at family meetings. On a few very notable occasions, not only did the patient's spouse come to the meeting, but the entire family showed up—grandparents, parents, brothers, sisters, children, and grandchildren—as well as friends, neighbors, and coworkers! So eager were these folks to help that they had already divvied up all of the household chores among themselves and were even bringing in cooked meals. The patients had had their lives taken away from them, had nothing to say about what was happening, and were left with nothing to do—except rebel. These patients fought against their families' theft of their lives and refused to do anything to manage their PPS. One patient actually went home from the meeting and started painting the house! These patients' internal emotional struggles with making lifestyle changes were short-circuited, replaced by an external battle with their families. These experiences lead to The Golden Rule for polio survivors' friends and families:

**KNOW EVERYTHING ABOUT PPS, SAY NOTHING, AND HELP
ONLY WHEN ASKED.**

Friends and family need to understand all about the cause and
treatment of PPS and help with physical chores, but only when
asked. Neither gentle reminders nor well-meaning nagging will
force polio survivors to eat breakfast, use a cane, take breaks, or
stop them from painting the house. Survivors must learn to ask
for help, take responsibility for caring for themselves, and
fashion a meaningful, albeit less active, new life on their own.

The Stress Mess

But how, after a lifetime of denying polio and using Type A
behavior to protect against "mortal danger," can polio survivors
face their fears and finally start caring for themselves? This is the
alpha and omega of the polio experience, the bottom line, the
final battle that must be waged and won if polio survivors are
going to manage PPS. But the problems seem too complicated,
too long-standing, and too deeply ingrained:

- There is a bedrock of Type A behavior that allowed polio
survivors to appear "normal" and reenter society—but that is
responsible for the overuse-abuse that triggers PPS.
- There is half a century of Type E programming that supposedly protected polio survivors from abuse, criticism by others,
and feeling like failures, but today prevents polio survivors from
caring for themselves and managing PPS.
- There's the double whammy of polio survivors having to
deal with shock and fear triggered by PPS at the same time they
are forced to confront the long-buried—or never addressed—
emotions associated with polio itself.
- And there's yet another Polio Paradox:

**POLIO SURVIVORS, WHOSE EARLY ABUSE BY THE MEDICAL
ESTABLISHMENT CAUSED A LIFELONG AVERSION TO
DOCTORS AND CARING FOR THEMSELVES, MUST NOW**

**TURN TO MEDICAL PROFESSIONALS TO HELP TREAT
AND MANAGE PPS.**

How can polio survivors fight old and new battles on so many fronts and have any chance of winning? How could anyone dig back through decades of painful emotions, dislodge entrenched behaviors, start listening to their bodies, entirely change their lifestyles, and change themselves mentally, emotionally, and physically?

Actually, it's more simple than it seems. It all boils down to this Polio Paradox:

**DESPITE CHEATING DEATH, CONQUERING DISABILITY, AND
OVERCOMING YEARS OF SEVERE PHYSICAL AND EMOTIONAL
PAIN TO BECOME THE BEST AND THE BRIGHTEST, POLIO
SURVIVORS BELIEVE THAT THEY HAVE NO RESOURCES THAT
WOULD ALLOW THEM TO BOTH MANAGE PPS *AND* SURVIVE.**

Polio survivors must reject this paradox and reclaim the truth: that all who had polio are survivors who have already proven they have the courage and internal resources to not only survive polio and PPS but also build a new life and even a better one.

So when it comes to managing PPS, there is only one issue: survival. And there is only one virulent process at the heart of the emotional and physical problems that underlie PPS and threatens survival: stress. If polio survivors can reject this Polio Paradox and annihilate stress, they can fight and win the physical and emotional battles with polio and PPS.

KNOWING THE ENEMY

One notion about stress may come from the same place as "Use it or lose it" and "No pain, no gain." It says that stress is actually good for you; that stress stimulates, activates, and motivates you; that life would be boring without stress. This idea that stress can be good is just plain wrong. Here's the real definition of stress:

STRESS IS YOUR BODY'S PHYSICAL AND EMOTIONAL RESPONSE WHEN IT THINKS YOU'RE ABOUT TO DIE!

That's right. Die. When your brain looks at what's happening in the world around you and decides that your life is at risk, your body is given two choices: fight or flight. You can either run away from whatever is trying to kill you or attack and vanquish it. In either case, your brain turns on the stress response system that is hardwired into your brain and body. Your nervous system goes into overdrive. Your muscles get tight so that they can contract quickly and forcefully. Adrenaline is released to make your heart pump faster and harder, pushing blood into your muscles and away from your skin. Your hands get clammy and cold; you feel jittery and anxious as you wait to fight or take flight.

If the threat to your life disappears, if you fight and eliminate it or successfully escape, your stress response system turns off. You feel exhausted, having used up tremendous amounts of energy, and go into rest mode to repair any damage and restore your body's energy reserves.

But what happens when the threat to your life doesn't disappear, but you can neither fight nor take flight? What happens when you got polio and it didn't go away, when you were torn from the safety of your parents and your home and hospitalized for months or years? What happens when you had years of painful physical therapy and surgery? What happens when you were abused by the very people who were supposed to be caring for you and learned that, in order to be safe in the world, you would have to appear "normal" and care for everyone except yourself?

What happens is that you became Type A in order to survive, and your stress system never turned off. You live every day with your stress response turned on, with feelings of anxiety, trouble falling asleep because your mind is racing, muscle spasms, and eventually the fatigue, muscle weakness, and pain that are PPS.

TURNING OFF THE TYPE A SWITCH

What then must you do to turn off the stress response system and treat your PPS? You have to take yourself out of overdrive and change your Type A ways. But if you believe that being Type A is the only way you can survive, why would you ever change? Because you have to change to manage your PPS. The first step on this road requires a leap of faith, a leap over the first Polio Paradox, and believing this:

BECAUSE OF EVERYTHING YOU HAVE SURVIVED, YOU WILL SURVIVE—AND THRIVE—IF YOU MAKE THE CHANGES NECESSARY TO MANAGE PPS.

To make this leap you need to look at the broad scope of your life, at the panorama of your own personal history. Polio survivors need to read these two words again and again and take in the depth and breadth of their full meaning:

POLIO
SURVIVOR

If you can remember all you have survived and appreciate how you have thrived *in spite* of polio, there can be no question that you have the ability to make the physical and emotional changes necessary to survive and thrive with PPS.

More than one patient has angrily asked me, "Do you expect me to change my entire personality and the way I live overnight?" My answer is always the same: "Yes . . . and no." If you can identify all of the things that trigger PPS, you can stop doing them and physically feel better virtually overnight. But the paradox here is that becoming less Type A will make you feel much better *physically* and sometimes much worse *emotionally*. And how could this not be true? If you believe that being Type A and doing for others has kept you alive all these years, changing your ways will surely get you killed. You will be violating the prime directive, the fundamental Polio Fiction:

IF I TAKE CARE OF MYSELF I WILL SURELY DIE!

Says Margo from chapter 7:

I have two personalities: the abused polio child and Superwoman! I would work fourteen-hour days doing my own work and then other people's work. . . . I developed this super Type A personality so I wouldn't be abandoned again and rejected like when I had polio. But it has ruined me.

It's crucial to replace this Polio Fiction and superperson lifestyle with this most important Post-Polio Precept:

DO UNTO YOURSELF AS YOU HAVE BEEN DOING FOR OTHERS.

When we begin treating a new patient we make "The Deal." We tell our patients that as they start doing for themselves they will quickly feel much better physically but feel worse emotionally. Why would anyone agree to such a deal? Because there isn't any other way. Post-polio pioneer and polio survivor Nancy Frick says, "The only thing worse than dealing with PPS is not dealing with it. To get from one side of a swamp to the other you have to get your feet wet. It's the only way to become a 'new' polio survivor." So here are some tips on making it across the swamp and becoming a "new" polio survivor (and not getting caught in jaws of the alligators).

Becoming a New Polio Survivor

Becoming a new polio survivor begins the moment you take that leap of faith and accept that you are indeed a survivor. Unfortunately, polio survivors can easily leap back just as they are about to enter the swamp when they encounter three of the "Four Emotional Horsemen" of PPS: denial, anger, and fear.

Denial, the Sand, and the Seesaw

Denial is not an unusual response in anyone who starts to experience new physical symptoms. But in some polio survivors denial has been raised to an art form. Remember that 25 percent of polio survivors in our 1985 Survey said they didn't think of themselves as being disabled before PPS appeared. So when PPS symptoms rear their ugly heads, polio survivors sometimes stick their heads deeply in the sand, giving themselves more and more to deny as PPS gets worse.

But there's usually a point when polio survivors run out of energy, run out of muscle strength, and run out of sand. When their heads come up and they look around, they don't like what they see. When the reality of new symptoms sets in and it becomes clear that functional abilities are ebbing away, polio survivors will seesaw between denial of PPS and anger or fear: anger that their bodies are no longer able to do what they had done and fear that they will be abused and rejected if they can no longer do what they are "supposed" to do.

The denial–fear/anger seesaw can go on for years while polio survivors continue to overuse neurons, lose function, and refuse to seek treatment. It's during this time that some polio survivors get on the Internet and read everything there is to be found about PPS. Some will even attend post-polio conferences, where they sit in the back of the room, speak to no one, and take in what information they can tolerate. Each year we have a Polio Update conference, where we talk about the cause and treatment of PPS. Patients have told me that they've had to attend Polio Updates as many as five times before they could summon the courage to come in for an evaluation. One of our patients came in to be evaluated six times in eighteen months before agreeing to be treated. Unfortunately, by the time he was ready for treatment his arms were too weak to allow him to continue working. The price for riding the seesaw can be very high.

When patients do come to The Post-Polio Institute they are often still on the seesaw, denying that they really need to see us and afraid of what they're going to hear. Those who were abused when they were young and have not seen a doctor for the past forty years—let alone been inside a hospital—are even more frightened and skeptical, wondering if they're going to be abused yet again. Some patients angrily demand to be convinced that PPS are real, that the poliovirus did do lasting damage to their bodies, that polio in fact set the stage for the symptoms they are experiencing today.

When polio survivors get off the seesaw, some just cry. They're tired of wasting what little energy they have denying with their minds what their bodies know to be true. They're tired of being tired and weak and in pain. But more than anything else, they cry because they're tired of their own denial and fear. They're exhausted by decades of keeping the "shameful secret" of their polio and the new secret of PPS. They cry because they're relieved that a door has been opened and that they finally can stop being "normal" and become who they really are: polio survivors.

DUCK AND COVER

When patients begin at The Post-Polio Institute, they receive medical and psychophysiological evaluations and list their goals. Most times the goals themselves are paradoxical, patients wanting to feel better while doing everything they did the same way they've been doing it. We talk right up front about changing from the "use it or lose it" philosophy to the "conserve to preserve" lifestyle. We discuss how lifestyle changes and assistive devices—canes, crutches, braces, and wheelchairs—are simply tools, means to an end, the end being conserving the remaining poliovirus-damaged neurons in order to stop the progression of PPS and actually decrease or eliminate new symptoms.

But it's here that fear and denial ride in again, as some polio survivors begin to duck the issue, telling me that they don't need to change their lifestyles or use any assistive device because:

"I don't do so much."
"I don't work too hard."
"I don't walk that far."

Our response to these feints is to discuss patients' symptoms, the symptoms' triggers, and point out the obvious: If polio survivors had been doing what was good for their bodies, they wouldn't have PPS. We also explain that polio survivors usually underestimate how much they really do and describe our 1997 study, which found that the more symptoms polio survivors have when they come to us for evaluation, the more symptoms they have after they graduate from the program. The fewer and less severe the PPS symptoms, and the sooner they are treated, the more likely it is that symptoms will decrease or disappear. The worse symptoms are when polio survivors agree to treatment, the more likely it is that permanent damage has been done.

Other polio survivors cover their fear with bluster, saying they won't change their lifestyles or use any assistive device because:

"I will not give in!"
"I'll change when I'm ready."
"I'll depend on a cane when there's no other choice."
"I'll be confined to a wheelchair when my muscles
become totally paralyzed."

Given their pasts, of course polio survivors aren't going to want to do less and look more disabled. Of course they've been programmed never to "give in." But when polio survivors say they won't give in, we suggest that giving in and managing PPS is better than giving up their ability to function. If polio survivors change only when they're "ready," if they use a cane when there's "no other choice," they've given their neurons no other choice but to fail. If polio survivors want to wait to change until they're "ready," wait until their muscles are paralyzed, they will have given up both their bodies and their lives.

IT IS BETTER TO LOOK GOOD THAN TO FEEL GOOD

Robert Louis Stevenson was right when he said, "Man is a creature who lives not upon bread alone, but principally by catchwords." Unfortunately, polio survivors get caught by the same words that trap everyone, such as *wheelchair-dependent, wheelchair-bound,* and *confined to a wheelchair.* The wheelchair remains the most frightening icon of polio, *the* symbol of disability, of incompetence, of invalidism. Over the years five patients have actually told me they would rather kill themselves than use a cane. How much less would polio survivors be expected to happily embrace a wheelchair?

Using a wheelchair does exact an emotional price. Our 1997 study found that polio survivors who used wheelchairs felt lonelier, less acceptable, and less worthwhile as members of society and as members of their own families. So one of our jobs at The Post-Polio Institute is to help polio survivors see that wheelchairs—and canes, braces, and crutches—are merely tools, means to the end of saving both poliovirus-damaged neurons and quality of life. When polio survivors refuse to consider using a wheelchair, I ask them why they use a car. They splutter and say it would take too much time and energy to walk everywhere without a car. And that's the reason to use a wheelchair: to use less time and energy to get from place to place, to be not wheelchair-dependent but wheelchair-*independent.*

Another concern expressed by polio survivors who can walk is that people will think it strange if they use a wheelchair and then stand up. Granted, it's expected that someone who uses a wheelchair isn't able to stand. But again, drivers do get out of their cars when they get where they're going. Why shouldn't wheelchair users?

We recommend having a pocket full of catchwords to explain whatever assistive device you use, depending on the situation and the audience. If a good friend asks about your wheelchair or other device, you can give the full explanation about polio and PPS. If an acquaintance or well-meaning observer asks why you're using a wheelchair or cane, you can respond with a simple

"I had polio," or the less revealing "I have a bad hip," or even "old football injury," "war wound," or "skiing accident." Of course, you always have the right to say, "That's not an appropriate question for you to ask." Along the same line, if you walk, use a wheelchair only to go long distances, and someone stares or comments when they see you stand up, you can always look down at the wheelchair, look back at the person, look up at heaven, and shout "It's a miracle!" and then go about your business. Or you can ignore them completely. Remember: It's your body and it's your life. You don't owe an explanation to anyone but yourself.

A Fiction That's Also a Fact

When faced with having to change their lives, some patients' fallback position is yet another Post-Polio Fiction:

**I DON'T NEED TO CHANGE BECAUSE THERE'S NOTHING
I CAN'T DO IF I PUT MY MIND TO IT!**

Unfortunately, this statement is very powerful because it isn't always fiction. Polio survivors are not like those who have had a stroke or a spinal cord injury, who immediately become unable to walk and who have no choice but to use canes, braces, or wheelchairs. Polio survivors' lives have been examples of "mind over matter." There has been nothing, absolutely *nothing*, that polio survivors couldn't do when they put their minds to it. But now, although the mind is more than willing, the body is becoming weak, and polio survivors are confronted with another Polio Paradox:

**THE MORE POLIO SURVIVORS BEND THEIR BODIES TO THEIR
WILL, THE LESS THEIR BODIES WILL BEND AND THE MORE
QUICKLY THEY WILL BREAK.**

When our patients agree to bend so that they won't break, to give in instead of give up, we extend our hands and offer to take the next step and go with them into the swamp.

Of Alligators and Anxiety

With both trepidation and hope, the six- to eight-week Post-Polio Institute program begins. A treatment plan is created based on patients' symptoms and goals. Patients meet weekly with their team—dietitian, psychotherapist, physical and occupational therapists—and begin daily logs of symptoms and the activities that trigger them (I'll explain the logs in the next chapter). The logs are the first alligator that patients encounter because they don't want to take time away from things they "should" be doing to fill them out. Some patients think they're getting worse when they do the logs because they see, in black and white, how severe and pervasive some PPS symptoms are. But despite how bothersome the logs are, patients tell us they are the single most helpful part of the program exactly because they are forced to see that they in fact do too much and walk too far each day, that their bodies do indeed need a break.

Once patients identify PPS triggers and start making changes to manage PPS, two other alligators rise out of the swamp: anxiety and guilt.

FLASHBACKS AND MOVING FORWARD

Anxiety sometimes arises when polio survivors merely enter The Institute. Some of our patients report disturbing and frightening dreams and flashbacks about their early polio experiences. A few have had panic attacks when they entered a physical therapy gym for the first time in forty years, while others thought they saw children they knew being treated for polio. Still other polio survivors recall abuse they hadn't thought about in decades or that they hadn't remembered:

To deal with PPS I not only have had to change my whole lifestyle and face the fear of dealing with a second disability, but also I have had to deal with many painful memories from the initial onset of the polio as a child, some terrible memories that I had repressed.

MARGO, CLASS OF '53

When memories of abuse do surface, patients sometimes question whether the events really happened or actually were as terrible as their memories or feelings suggest. Some ask whether they should undergo hypnosis or even drug-induced memory recovery to be certain about what happened to them. We have found that the specific details of painful early experiences are not important. It is only important that patients recognize and express their feelings about painful past events. This is where psychotherapy becomes central to the treatment of PPS: to support polio survivors through what can be terrifying days and nights; help them understand the origin of their anxiety, panic, and flashbacks; learn to tolerate these feelings and continue treatment in spite of them.

Painful memories can actually be helpful, proving to patients that they are indeed survivors. There is tremendous strength to be found in the knowledge that those who had polio in fact survived even the worst kinds of abuse, that they are no longer children but competent adults who can indeed protect themselves from anyone who might try to hurt them, and that they have the emotional strength to stare down the anxiety and change their lives to deal with PPS.

A SELF-CARE PHOBIA

Anxiety and even panic attacks can also arise when polio survivors stop being Type A, stop doing for others, and start taking care of themselves. Another way of looking at this kind of anxiety is that polio survivors actually have a self-care phobia. One treatment for phobias is called implosion, in which an individual agrees to face the cause of the anxiety. For example, when individuals who are claustrophobic force themselves to get inside an elevator, their anxiety builds to a crescendo—then fades away as they discover that being closed in doesn't kill them. We use similar but much milder techniques with our patients. At the beginning of treatment we ask patients to agree to at least try things that cause anxiety—using a brace or crutches, taking a rest break, asking others for help—or stop doing the things that they think they "should" do and say no to others. Once polio survivors discover that they do not die when they appear more disabled, start taking care of themselves, and even ask others for help, their anxiety decreases and even disappears. That's why we recommend that patients stay away from anti-anxiety medications unless they are having frequent panic attacks or are so anxious that they can't participate in therapy. Anxiety can actually help uncover roadblocks to self-care.

THE GIFT OF GUILT

Even more than anxiety, the emotion that prevents polio survivors from changing their lives is guilt. Guilt kicks in when polio survivors stop being Type E, stop doing "everything for everybody every minute of every day." What is guilt? Guilt is your mother's—or father's, or society's—voice inside your head telling you what you "should" do to be acceptable, what you "should" do if you are going to survive. Type E polio survivors live their lives by dozens of "shoulds":

"I should do whatever anyone wants whenever they want it."
"I should be in control of myself and everything else."
"I should always be doing something and never rest."
"I should be perfect in everything I do."

I've borrowed this Post-Polio Precept from a sign that hung in the office of psychotherapist Fritz Perls:

THOU SHALT NOT "SHOULD" ON THYSELF.

Guilt, just like anxiety, fuels the phobia that stops you from taking care of yourself. The less you do what you "should," the more you say no to others, the more guilt you feel and the less you will want to say no.

But believe it or not guilt, and even anxiety, can be a gift. I know that's hard to accept, but think about it. These extremely unpleasant emotions provide you with a kind of built-in biofeedback. If you don't feel guilt or anxiety, you must be doing what you've always done—not take care of yourself. When you feel guilty or anxious, you must be staring down your fears, changing your life, and managing your PPS. This notion is the origin of the most important emotional Post-Polio Precept for managing PPS:

IF YOU'RE NOT GUILTY AND ANXIOUS, YOU'RE NOT TAKING CARE OF YOURSELF, YOU'RE NOT TREATING YOUR PPS, AND YOU'RE NOT BECOMING A "NEW" POLIO SURVIVOR.

Why would you choose to plod through this swamp, intentionally causing yourself to feel anxious and guilty? Because, as Nancy Frick says, the only way to the other side of the swamp is through it. What no one has ever told you is that while stress burns *you* out, anxiety and guilt burn *themselves* out. The more you can tolerate anxiety and guilt, the more you will be able to care for yourself, and the less anxiety and guilt you'll feel.

Of course, the trick is tolerating anxiety and guilt during the first few weeks of taking care of yourself. Here again is where psychotherapy is so important: it helps our patients make it all the way across the swamp. And it is a hard slog. Janet had trouble staying the course. She would sometimes use only one of her two short leg braces, and sometimes none at all. She sometimes refused to keep logs or pace activities. She would use a cane some days, and try to walk a mile without it on others:

I didn't want to look disabled or even think to myself that I had polio or have PPS. And I didn't want to appear selfish, like I was not pulling my weight. The more I did physically the less time I had to feel, the less afraid and guilty I was, but the more symptoms I had. I literally ran— well, walked—away from my feelings. I didn't stop until I hit the proverbial brick wall. And when I hit it, I tried to climb over it! It's like I was physically running away from people who were going to abuse me.

Usually it's the "voices" in polio survivors' heads, not what family, friends, and coworkers are actually saying or doing, that say it's selfish to save one's own body and quality of life. We ask patients to think about the definition of *selfish:* when you do for yourself without thinking about anyone else. *Selfless* is when you do for everyone else without thinking about yourself—being Type E. *Self-centered* is when you choose what you're going to do after you've thought about your own needs and wants as well as considering others'.

When polio survivors go from being selfless and Type E to being self-centered, they automatically think they have become totally selfish. But as they redefine themselves as self-centered, guilt fades away. Patients discard the "Good Chart," become able to care for themselves and begin to believe and act like they can have both self-worth *and* PPS. They discover that their Type A and Type E ways have been more a habit than a necessity for survival. It is wonderful to watch patients take care of themselves despite guilt and anxiety, and come out on the other side of the swamp feeling better both physically and emotionally.

THE RETURN OF THE FIRST 'GATOR

Unfortunately, there's a problem when polio survivors emerge from the swamp feeling better. The first alligator returns. Sometimes it's not helpful for polio survivors to feel better, because some go back to denying that they have PPS at all. They once again do all the Type A things they'd done before and PPS symptoms return as they again ride the post-polio roller coaster: overdoing, crashing, recovering, and then overdoing again.

Sometimes our patients intentionally test their limits, to see whether they really need to take care of themselves, to prove that they really have PPS. Other times patients make a conscious choice to use their energy and risk increasing symptoms—and possibly sacrificing some neurons—to do something physically taxing. And that's okay. After all, the fundamental tenet of The Post-Polio Institute program is for polio survivors to turn off their autopilot and decide for themselves what they're going to do with their energy, their muscle strength, and their remaining motor neurons.

To encourage patients to stay off the roller coaster and to help them make good choices, we ask them to continue to keep daily logs between graduation from the treatment program and their first follow-up meeting with the team one month later. At all the follow-up meetings—one, three, six, and twelve months after graduation—the team reviews the patients' goals and symptoms, continues to monitor any new problems and discusses how to manage them.

For many if not most polio survivors, dealing with PPS will be the most difficult battle they will ever wage, even more difficult than fighting polio itself. Sadly, it is a battle that some polio survivors will not be able to join. As I mentioned, 12 percent of our patients leave the program, overwhelmed by anxiety and guilt, the fear of looking disabled, and the fear of being abused again. When this happens, we keep the door open, hoping they will return. But only 10 percent of all patients who have refused or left treatment have returned to The Post-Polio Institute, typically about four years later, and always in much worse shape than we first met them. Even more unfortunate, 80 percent of those who return refuse treatment or quit again! It will be no surprise to you that these patients are 25 percent more Type A and 20 percent more sensitive to criticism and failure than patients who complete treatment.

Fortunately, the overwhelming majority of polio survivors are able to fight and to win the battle. However, even when the battle is won, the last Horseman remains.

THE FOURTH HORSEMAN

Once you've disposed of the first three Horsemen, after you've discarded denial and once anxiety and guilt burn away, all that's left is the emotion with which we began: sadness. As I said up front, if you weren't sad about having PPS—about losing hard-won functional abilities, about changing your personality, your relationships with nearly everyone in your life, and the way you do absolutely everything—you would be crazy. Patients will cry the most at the beginning of treatment and at the end. At the beginning they're frightened and tired; at the end they're sad. Patients sometimes don't know why they cry as they're ready to graduate. More than one patient has said, "I feel so much better. My family is being so helpful. Even my boss understands. I should not be crying."

This is the last "should" polio survivors need to discard. Polio survivors have every reason to cry, about what happened to them years ago and about what's happening to them now. Here again, sadness is not depression and no antidepressant will—or should—stop this genuine feeling of loss, of grief. Many patients have asked me, "What good is crying?" I always reply, "What good is laughing?" Tears and laughter are expressions of genuine emotions; they are ends in themselves. You know you've become a new polio survivor when you care enough about yourself, are self-centered and so in touch with what you feel—physically and emotionally—that you are able to cry and truly feel this Post-Polio Precept:

GRIEF IS A RELIEF.

Patients say they shouldn't grieve because it's a sign they're feeling sorry for themselves. Well, feeling sorry is just fine. Everyone has a right to feel sorry for their losses and about the things that have hurt them. I think everyone should feel sorry, sad, grieve, and even cry for at least five minutes every morning. After all, there are only four basic emotions: fear and anger, sadness and joy. Many polio survivors have spent so much time and energy fending off the first three, and making sure others feel the last, there has been no time or energy left for their *own* joy. And one joy in particular that has been left far behind, and sometimes not experienced at all, is one of the greatest emotional and physical joys of all.

Becoming a Sexy Polio Survivor

For those of you who've been surfing the Internet, you may have noticed the phenomenal amount of information about sex on disability sites. Yes, unbridled, undiluted, and unimpeded discussions about sex—fears and frustrations, fetters and fulfillment—among people with all kinds of disabilities, from high-level quads to quadruple amputees. Yet on the post-polio sites you'll find almost no mention of that three-letter four-letter word. I guess this shouldn't be a surprise. Most of our patients don't mention sex either, and there are several reasons why:

- Polio survivors grew up in the 1940s and 1950s, when discussing sex was the same as walking down Main Street without your clothes.
- Fifty years ago, even more than today, people with disabilities were thought not to be fully human, let alone sexual beings.
- It was also crucial back in the dark ages that anything not "normal" be hidden.

So if polio survivors expected to have a relationship with someone their disability had to be hidden. Since the physical effects of polio were often hard to hide, bodies were covered and polio was ignored or even denied. I've mentioned that some of our patients have never admitted even to their spouses that they'd had polio.

The process of covering, denying, or ignoring the reality of your own body causes problems. Some polio survivors turned off any awareness of their bodies below the neck, since the principal feelings from down below were often weakness and pain. But since you can't turn off pain without turning off pleasure as well, turning off feelings will make sensuality or sexuality nearly impossible, or as appealing as eating dry toast. Some polio survivors have turned off all feelings, both below and above the neck. Walling off your feelings cuts off the ability to be intimate with yourself and with others. And intimacy is the gateway to sexuality. Of course polio survivors who were abused will be much less likely to risk intimacy. And when abused polio survivors begin to use braces, crutches, and wheelchairs again, painful memories of the past and the reality of disability can no longer be hidden. Old fears of unacceptability and new fears of rejection surface and cut sexuality off at the pass.

"IF YOU THINK YOU'RE SEXY"

One of the first Internet disability bulletin boards was called "Sex Is 99% Mental." It's true. Sexy is as sexy thinks. Sure, you may not look like Cindy Crawford or Mel Gibson. But how many people do? What counts is how you feel about yourself. If you're not acceptable to yourself, you won't be acceptable to, intimate with, or sexually available to anyone else.

The first step to intimacy and sexuality is everything discussed above: recognizing and dealing with the emotional reality of polio, of any abuse you experienced because of it, and of PPS. You then need to identify your own negative feelings about your body and stop projecting them into the heads of spouses, friends, and lovers. And if you've turned off your body to stop feeling physical pain, you need to reopen communication and experience good physical feelings. Once you have decreased your post-polio fatigue, muscle weakness, and pain, you need to start sending pleasant physical sensation to your brain. Start out with long, luxurious baths, a whirlpool, or—best of all—a massage. When you make nice to your body and good feelings start traveling up to your head, other good physical sensations, even erotic ones, will follow along up that stairway (or ramp) to paradise.

When all is said and done, when you're with your spouse or a partner to whom you're attracted and feel comfortable, there's a simple Golden Rule for being an intimate and sexy polio survivor:

TURN OFF YOUR HEAD, TURN ON YOUR BODY, AND JUST DO IT!

From Head to Toe

Once you've escaped the Horsemen, the alligators, and made it through the swamp, the mechanics of managing PPS are easy. It's actually kind of like carpentry: a brace to shore up a weak leg here, a cane to take the weight off there. Once you've remodeled your head and shored up your body, though, will there always be smooth sailing? To be honest, no. Your body and your life will always have ups and downs, both emotional and physical. When you feel better you'll probably take a ride or two on the roller coaster. Like some of our patients, you may stick the cane in a closet for a week to test your limits or to prove you don't really have PPS. But then you'll use it again. Guilt and fear will nip at your heels. And from time to time each of the Horsemen will ride in for a visit.

But knowledge of what's happening in your head and in your body is ultimately the power that will conquer PPS. If you have learned what your body needs, learned to say no to others and to the "voices" in your own head—and learned to be self-centered—you'll know how to get off the roller coaster, how to get away from the alligators, and how to tell the Horsemen to ride on by. But as perfect as so many polio survivors have always been at everything, try not to add more stress to your life by wanting to be a perfect, nonstressed, always self-centered, "new" polio survivor. Over time, making choices and dealing with the physical and emotional reality of PPS will become your natural way of life. The last question we need to answer is what that way of life must be.

CHAPTER 16

Less Is More: Managing PPS

I've done things I never thought I would have to do. I started using crutches all the time and slowed my life down. I got two long leg braces. My friends thought I'd grown taller because I was no longer stooped over. Then I did something I never thought I would want to do: I got a wheelchair. All of this was emotionally hard, very hard. It's still is. But the quality of my entire life has improved. Weakness, fatigue, pain . . . they almost disappear when I take care of myself. I haven't felt this good in twenty years.

GARY, CLASS OF '48

Finally, we can put all the pieces together. You now know more than any doctor you're likely to meet about what polio did to your body and the state of your post-polio spinal cord and brain. You know all there is to know about the cause of PPS—and you also know that there is no magic pill, no exercise regimen, that will make new symptoms disappear. You have learned what can be done to treat problems as different as cold intolerance, sleep apnea, nighttime muscle twitching, and hypoglycemia. And most importantly, you know the mental pitfalls that could prevent you

from dealing with PPS at all. So the final question is what can
be done for PPS symptoms that can't be treated, that require
something other than breathing machines or medication,
polypropylene socks or protein.

That "something other" is symptom management. Management, even more than treatment, is the bulwark, the *sine qua non*,
the principal means to the ultimate end of feeling better now and
preventing the progression of PPS. When we talk to our patients
about managing PPS, we use the analogy of diabetes. Diabetes
can't be cured, and while its symptoms can be decreased or eliminated—and long-term damage may be prevented—by taking
medication, even more important is being aware of symptoms,
decreasing stress, eating properly, and monitoring blood sugar. It
might be helpful to think of PPS as "diabetes of the neurons." PPS
can't be cured, and while its symptoms can be decreased or eliminated—and long-term damage may be prevented—by taking
some medications, what's critical is being aware of symptoms,
decreasing stress, eating properly, and sometimes even monitoring blood sugar. So the first and most important step in managing PPS is this Post-Polio Precept:

LISTEN TO YOURSELF.

Polio survivors are more sensitive than even the most sophis-
ticated computerized equipment in determining their own levels
of muscle weakness, pain, and fatigue. You need to be able to
identify when you're having a symptom and what's triggering it
before you can get rid of the trigger and the symptom.

Listening to their bodies is one of the most difficult things
polio survivors can do. I've talked about the varieties of physical
and emotional pain that survivors have experienced throughout
their lives. And I've noted that one common response to this pain
was polio survivors turning off any awareness of their bodies and
any feelings they had below the neck. Many polio survivors have
been sending orders to their bodies for forty years without listening for so much as a "Yes, sir!" So the experience of listening
to your body will be new, difficult, and even frightening, espe-

cially when the messages you first get back are weakness, fatigue, and pain.

Because listening is so fundamental, the most powerful tool in treating PPS is the daily log.

Each day our patients write down how well and how long they slept, what they ate and when, and all the activities they did throughout the day: bathing, dressing, climbing stairs, standing, walking, working, cleaning, shopping, and driving. Next to each activity patients rate their exertion using the six-to-twenty scale; they also note locations and severity of muscle weakness and pain, as well as severity of fatigue, difficulty breathing and swallowing, on a scale from none through severe. Patients also wear a pedometer (a device that measures steps) on the hip over their shorter leg, writing down their steps next to each activity and total steps at the end of the day.

At the end of each day patients review the logs and pick two activities that produced symptoms. They note what they felt ("Both legs severely weak"), what they were doing ("Stood ironing for sixty minutes"), and how they could change the activity to eliminate symptoms ("Get spouse to do ironing!").

Before completing the daily logs, most patients have no idea how much they do in a day, which activities trigger symptoms, and how badly they feel throughout the day. Our patients have also found that there's a "symptom gap"—doing too much on one day may not trigger symptoms until the next day, or even the day after that.

Patients also have no idea how far they walk each day and the relationship between walking and their symptoms. Kathy McCullough, chief occupational therapist at The Post-Polio Institute, collected a dozen sets of daily logs from our most compliant patients—those who followed all of the self-care recommendations made by the treatment team. The logs were kept for the six weeks or so during which they were treated and for the month after graduation before they returned for their first follow-up meeting with the team. Kathy compiled the total number of steps each day, along with the patients' maximum ratings for exertion, fatigue, muscle weakness, and pain. We used this infor-

Name: **Day:**   **Date:**

Time	Activities & Steps	Perceived Exertion	Muscle Weakness	Overall Fatigue	Pain Mood	
		RATE: mild — moderate — severe				Symptoms:
Up	Food:					
	Sleep Quality?:					What did you do?
						How did you do it?
Break	Snack?:					How could you change?
Noon	Food:					
						Symptoms:
						What did you do?
Break	Snack?:					How did you do it?
6 pm	Food:					How could you change?
	Total Steps:					

Exertion Scale:

6	7	8	9	10	11	12	13	14	15	16	17	18	19	20
Very, Very Light		Very Light		Fairly Light			Somewhat Hard		Hard		Very Hard		Very, Very Hard	

DAILY LOG

mation to see what the relationships were among number of steps each day, exertion, and PPS symptoms.

On average, the patients entered the program walking twenty-five hundred steps each day, almost half a mile. Patients rated their average maximum exertion as a twelve, or "somewhat hard," with maximum fatigue, muscle weakness, and pain rated as "moderate." At the one-month follow-up, patients had reduced their total number of daily steps to eighteen hundred, were rating their maximum exertions as a ten, or between "very light" and "fairly light," and their maximum fatigue, muscle weakness, and pain as "mild to moderate." We calculated that, for patients' daily ratings of fatigue, muscle weakness, and pain to have been "mild," they would have had to reduce the number of steps they were walking when they began the program by 20 percent.

If you'd like, make copies of the form and keep the daily log for one week. At the end of the week add together your total number of daily steps and plug them into this formula to calculate how many steps you need to take to minimize your PPS symptoms:

$$(\textit{Total Number of Steps for the Week}) \times 0.8$$

When you've reduced your daily steps, identified your symptoms, and noted their triggers, you've begun to apply the next Post-Polio Precept:

CONSERVE TO PRESERVE.

Even though you were told by your doctors and physical therapists to "use it or lose it" when you were recovering from the polio attack, you need to be aware of this Polio Paradox:

THE EXTREME EXERCISES AND THERAPIES THAT HELPED POLIO SURVIVORS TO APPEAR "NORMAL" SET THE STAGE FOR PPS AND ARE THE *OPPOSITE* OF WHAT YOU NEED TO DO TODAY TO MANAGE PPS.

You know now that all of the hard-driving physical therapy polio survivors did after the polio attack caused muscle fibers to get too big and neurons to sprout too much. The time has come to do an about-face. You need to conserve energy to preserve your neurons by applying these Post-Polio Precepts, beginning with:

STOP BEFORE YOU START.

We ask our patients to begin conserving by stopping all activities they don't absolutely have to do during their first month of treatment. We ask them only to get up, get dressed, do the work they must do, come home, and rest in the evenings. We ask patients to ask family members and friends to take over all energy-depleting activities at least for that month, like shopping, laundry, and cleaning. We ask that patients postpone extraordinary jobs, such as cleaning the gutters or work-related travel, and to put extracurricular activities—evening meetings, physical therapy, swimming or other exercise they may be doing—on hold.

Once patients start to rest, their PPS symptoms quickly decrease as they reach their baseline. Once logs identify and patients eliminate activities that trigger symptoms, we ask them to slowly reintroduce activities, one at a time, in ways that do not increase symptoms, and to apply this Post-Polio Precept:

BRAKE BEFORE YOU BREAK.

Physiatrist Jim Agre found that polio survivors who paced activity—that is, worked and then rested for at least an equal amount of time—could do 240 percent more work with fewer symptoms than if they pushed themselves straight through to the finish. This is why taking two fifteen-minute rest breaks per day—that's doing absolutely *nothing* for fifteen minutes midmorning and midafternoon—is so important. But remember, if you rest because you're fatigued, weak, or in pain, you've stopped too late to protect your neurons and aren't following this Post-Polio Precept.

And whether you're working, recreating, or taking a break, this Precept is an important energy saver:

DON'T STAND WHEN YOU CAN SIT, AND DON'T SIT WHEN YOU CAN LIE DOWN.

Place chairs strategically around your home and office. Get a bench for the shower; sit to shave or apply makeup; get a high stool with a back support to work in the kitchen. And make sure any seat is high enough so that you can easily get up once you sit down. Low, cushy chairs make your legs and arms work too hard when you go to stand up. So does a low toilet. Getting a toilet booster seat having a frame with grab bars, so that it's easier to push yourself up and off the throne, is a way to begin applying this next Post-Polio Precept:

WORK SMARTER, NOT HARDER.

Plan your day and week ahead of time by listing all the activities you need to do, including your breaks and meals. Plan activities by *place*, doing everything in one location before you move on to the next. It's not conserving or preserving to get up in the morning, go downstairs for coffee, go upstairs to shower, come downstairs to eat, go back upstairs to dress, and come down to go to work. If you plan ahead you can finish all your upstairs activities, then do downstairs activities so as to minimize trips and "trips" on the stairs. By the same token, if you have errands to do around town or even around the office, plan one trip that incorporates all the stops (with a short break between errands) instead of making many individual trips.

When you plan your day and week, also divide activities by *effort* into heavy and light (cooking may be light, for instance, and food shopping heavy) and alternate lighter and heavier jobs throughout the day and the week, never doing more than one heavy activity per day. Look at your logs and find your best time to do heavy work. If you have more energy in the morning or early in the week, do heavy tasks then, always followed by a break. Do fewer daytime activities, and no heavy ones, if you're planning a night on the town.

Even better, trade heavy jobs with someone else. You do the checkbook from now on and let your spouse do the shopping. Or just ask someone to do a heavy job for you. Asking for help is not a sign of "giving in" to polio or PPS. Let family members, neighbors, friends, and coworkers help with heavy jobs like laundry, shopping, cleaning, lifting, and carrying. Believe it or not, other people *like* to be helpful and feel needed. And believe it or not, asking for help on the job is a right granted to you by the Americans with Disabilities Act. That's right—there's a federal law that provides Americans with what's called "reasonable accommodation" to allow you to do the "essential functions" of your job despite a disability. You can actually ask your boss to have someone else run errands and do heavy lifting if these aren't activities your job requires. What's more, you can ask to lie down during your two fifteen-minute breaks, and for a thirty-minute lie-down at lunch. You can even ask to work from home one or more days a week, or to telecommute, if your duties permit.

Speaking of permit, you need to get a state "disabled driver" permit right away, and to use the "handicapped parking" spots every time you park. While you're out shopping, buy assistive devices that will help you conserve and preserve. Get a reacher to grab things off the floor or down from a high shelf, instead of bending, reaching, or climbing. Buy devices with wheels—a rolling kitchen cart, laundry basket, luggage carrier—so you can pull instead of lift and carry. And look for electric gadgets that will do the work for your muscles: electric can openers, mixers, and toothbrushes. Speaking of assistive devices, here's a powerful Post-Polio Precept:

A CRUTCH IS NOT A CRUTCH.

And a brace is not a sign of "giving in" to polio. As I mentioned, polio survivors don't want to "depend" on devices, wheelchairs being the most frightening icons of polio and disability. But crutches also have a negative connotation; our 1997 study found that our patients who used crutches felt less acceptable and worthwhile as family members. Polio survivors have often said to me:

> "I don't need an assistive device because I'm
> always very careful when I walk."
> "I don't need anything to help me walk because I
> hold on to the walls and furniture inside the house and
> on to my husband outside."

Well, here's a Post-Polio Precept your credenza, wallpaper, and spouse will appreciate:

WALLS, FURNITURE, AND SPOUSES ARE *NOT* ASSISTIVE DEVICES.

You need to be secure and independent in walking, not clinging for dear life to your couch or your spouse. Before you dismiss even considering using a brace or crutch, here are some important facts to consider. Polio survivors use three times less energy and actually look better when they walk using a brace on a weakened leg. What's more, PPS researcher Mary Klein measured leg and arm muscle strength in polio survivors over the course of a year and discovered what others have found: Polio survivors' thigh muscles and those that move your ankles up and down are getting weaker. But unexpectedly, she found that polio survivors' hip muscles—those that move your upper leg forward and prevent you from swaying from side to side when you walk, as well as those that pull your upper leg backward to help lock your knee when you stand—are also getting weaker. This weakness is due to hip muscles substituting for lower leg muscles that have always been weak. So it's not just your ankles and upper leg muscles that are getting weaker. *All* the muscles you use to walk and stand are tiring out and need assistance.

And if you think you won't fall because you're "always very careful" when you walk, here's a frightening finding. A survey of polio survivors found that more than 60 percent reported they had fallen within the past year. Of those who fell, about 60 percent needed medical attention, and just over one-third broke a bone. There's no such thing as being so careful that you won't fall.

THE NEW BRACES

One thing you need to know up front is that the braces available today are nothing like the heavy, clanking metal-and-leather devices of the 1950s. Today's braces are made of lightweight graphite, or of plastic that's molded to the shape of your leg and fit inside your shoe. When we first started treating polio survivors, many didn't even want to consider these new types of braces, even though they were less visible and so much lighter. Our patients felt safe with and were used to their old contraptions. They believed they couldn't walk in anything but the brace they'd been wearing for forty years.

Of the hundreds of braces we've prescribed, not even a handful of patients rejected or were dissatisfied with their new braces. Two graphite long leg braces turned Gary's life around. Here's a look at the new braces and what they can do for you:

• **Molded Ankle-Foot Orthosis (MAFO).** The MAFO, made of plastic molded to your lower leg, replaces the old double metal upright short leg brace that is the most common brace worn by polio survivors. The MAFO is one piece and looks like an L, with a foot plate that fits inside your shoe and an upright going up the back of your calf that's held in place with a Velcro strap. A MAFO can do several things. It can stop foot drop, preventing you from tripping on your toe, and protect the muscles that flex your hip, since you don't have to pull your leg up to clear your dropping foot. A MAFO can also push your knee backward to take the load off a weakened thigh muscle, and can give a spring to your step for those whose calf muscles are weak. But avoid MAFOs with a hinged ankle joint that prevents your foot from dropping but allows your ankle to bend upward. Hinged MAFOs do nothing to push the knee backward or to help spring you forward.

- **Knee-Ankle-Foot Orthosis (KAFO).** A KAFO also can be made of lightweight plastic molded to your lower and upper leg, or it can have graphite uprights. Both attach with Velcro straps and have a metal joint at the knee. There are two types of knee joints. The old familiar joint with drop locks prevents the knee from bending when you stand and walk. A newer development, the offset joint, can be used by polio survivors who have some strength in their quadriceps and whose knees bend backward just a bit. The offset joint doesn't lock but prevents the knee from bending when your leg is straight, so you can swing your leg normally when you walk but be secure when you're standing.

"Painless Posture"

Besides managing muscle weakness, braces, canes, and crutches reduce leg muscle, joint, and back pain. But you have to develop what we call "painless posture" in order to reap all the benefits these devices have to offer. If you can stand, get in front of a mirror and see how you look. Are you slumped when you stand with (a) head drooping, (b) shoulders humped, and (c) upper back curved forward? Is your head or body tilted to one side?

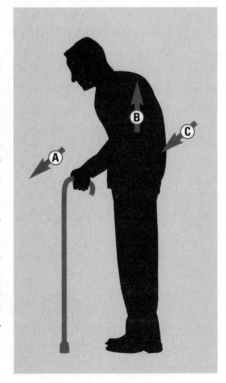

STANDING PAINFULLY

If you slump, droop, or tilt, you're putting tremendous strain on your back and neck muscles, which are not strong enough to continuously hold the weight of your head and upper body against the pull of gravity. These muscles will hurt and go into spasm if they continuously contract in order to prevent you from falling forward or toppling sideways. To manage pain in all of these muscles and joints, you need to apply this Post-Polio Precept:

MAKE GRAVITY YOUR FRIEND.

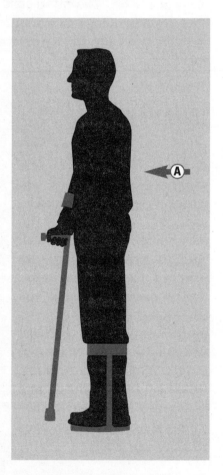

To make gravity your friend, you need to develop the key to painless posture, a lumbar lordosis (a)—that is, a slight curve in your lower back. You need to align your head, neck, chest, and legs so that gravity is pulling directly through the center of your body and you don't need your muscles to contract or spasm to prevent you from falling forward or from side to side:

If you tilt to one side or have a brace on one leg, a cane in the hand on the other side will take the load off weak muscles and stop you from tilting. If you have low back, belly, leg, or hip muscle weakness, you may need two forearm crutches to

STANDING PAINLESSLY

keep your body upright and to balance yourself from side to side. If one leg is shorter, a shoe lift will also help you become balanced.

And you need painless posture when walking as well as standing, when your muscles not only have to keep you upright but also must move your body forward. When you walk, try not to lead with your chin, your head, neck, and chest drooping forward. Try to walk with your head tucked straight backward like a turtle, your chin parallel to the floor. Look down with your eyes if you need to watch the ground for objects that could trip you. Granted, painless posture requires a lot of relearning, but it is worth the effort.

MERRILY YOU ROLL ALONG?

Most polio survivors who come to us are "underassisted," having thrown away canes, crutches, and braces decades ago. We typically recommend that polio survivors "trade up" to the next level of assistive device following this Post-Polio Precept:

IF YOU HAVE FOOT DROP AND DON'T USE A BRACE, YOU NEED ONE.
IF YOU HAVE ONE SHORT LEG BRACE, YOU ALSO NEED A CANE IN THE OPPOSITE HAND.
IF YOU HAVE A LONG LEG BRACE AND ARE USING A CANE, YOU NEED TWO FOREARM CRUTCHES.
IF YOU HAVE TWO BRACES AND ALREADY USE FOREARM CRUTCHES, YOU NEED TO ROLL INSTEAD OF WALK.

Yeah, I said roll. You knew we were going to have to come back to this. I've discussed the emotional reasons why polio survivors don't want to use a wheelchair. Here are some of the physical reasons why you should roll instead of walk. Even if you use two crutches plus a leg brace, you're still using those weakening hip muscles to move your legs forward. What's more, the weaker your legs, the more weight you put on canes or crutches, and the more strain you put on your hands, arms, and shoulders. Mary Klein found that the wrist, arm, and shoulder muscles you need to use a cane or crutch were losing about 15 percent of their strength per year, just over twice the rate of strength loss in leg muscles. You may need a brace plus a cane or crutches to take the load off your weakened leg muscles, but you also need some way to save your hip and arm muscles. How can you do that? By rolling instead of walking, especially outside the house and when you're going a distance.

Time for a Power Trip?

If you're still reading, I might as well take the big plunge. If rolling is better than walking for your leg and hip muscles, and if arm and shoulder muscles get weaker twice as fast as your legs, should you really be pushing a manual wheelchair? Whether you should push depends on how strong your arm and shoulder muscles are, how much endurance they have, and whether they're in pain. For those who shouldn't or can't push a manual wheelchair, we recommend lightweight power chairs, not scooters. Scooters aren't good if you have hand, arm, shoulder, neck, or upper back pain or weakness, since they have a T-bar tiller that forces you to hold your arms up and slump forward to steer. A power wheelchair with a joystick on the armrest allows you to drive with painless posture while sitting, arms at your sides and shoulders down, steering using only your hand, or even just your fingers. Still, one problem with all wheelchairs is that they have sling seats and backs that prevent you from sitting with painless posture.

Sitting Pretty

Painless posture is essential regardless of what you're sitting in. Notice how you're sitting right now. Are you slumped with (a) head drooping and (b) shoulders humped as you read with the

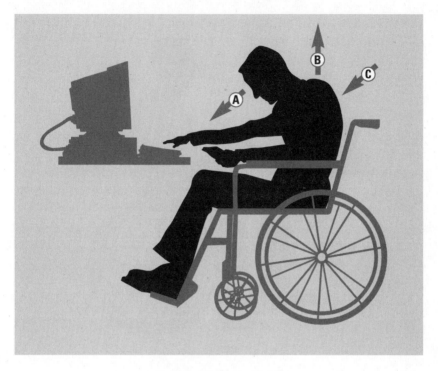

SITTING PAINFULLY

book in your lap and your upper back curved forward? Are you sitting unsupported with your back away from the chair (c)? Are you tilting your head or leaning your body to one side?

Take a look at the logs you've been keeping. Do you notice that neck, back, and headache pain increase the longer you sit, read, or work at the computer?

The key to sitting pretty is painless posture, starting with the same lumbar lordosis you need to be upstanding. Most chairs don't give you lumbar support to get the curve you need in your low back. Most chairs, as well as the standard wheelchair sling back, actually force you to bend forward and slump. For painless sitting posture, place your feet flat on the floor or on your wheelchair footrests, keep your knees bent at a ninety-degree angle, feet directly under your knees, and put your butt against the back of the chair.

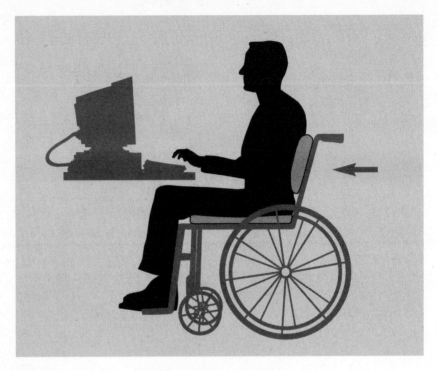

SITTING PAINLESSLY

Then place a lumbar cushion just above your belt line. As you lean back against the cushion, your low back curves, giving you a lumbar lordosis (arrow), and straightening your upper back, so that gravity is pulling through the center of your body. All you have to do then is make sure your head isn't tilting to one side, drop your shoulders, tuck your head, level your chin, and voilà, painless posture.

Any wheelchair sling back can be replaced with a removable rigid back that has foam inserts to provide adjustable back support and the right amount of lumbar curve. Solid backs with foam are available that can be custom-formed, if you have upper body weakness or scoliosis, to cradle and hold your body up if your muscles can't. If you have upper back or neck pain or muscle weakness, you may find that a shoulder-high or head-high back or headrest will allow your muscles to be supported and to relax. For those who aren't rolling, a lumbar cushion and high-backed chairs serve the same purpose.

It's also important that you're balanced and supported below the waist. If one buttock is smaller than the other, or if you have scoliosis and your upper body tilts to one side, an adjustable wheelchair cushion that has separate inflatable air bladders or foam inserts of different heights and firmness will lift one side of your pelvis and balance your body side to side, just as a shoe lift balances you from side to side if one leg is shorter. The Post-Polio Institute's famous "butt lifts," small wedges of specially cut foam, are placed under a small buttock to allow you to sit in any chair without tilting to one side. Those who don't use wheelchairs can buy lightweight foam cushions to provide a soft seat and add some height to chairs to make standing up easier.

Whether you're sitting or standing, there's another Post-Polio Precept to keep in mind:

DON'T FEED THE SPASMS.

Once you've attained painless posture, you need to make sure that you're not doing anything to feed the spasms—that is, being in any position that allows a muscle to shorten and contract more easily. If you tend to lean to one side in a chair or put your elbows on a chair's armrests, your neck and back muscles will shorten and can more easily spasm. Try not to use armrests at all; sit instead with your hands in your lap. When you're at a table, it's best if you put your legs completely underneath, with your belly touching its edge, so you're not bending forward or forced to hold yourself up with your elbows. You can raise a table or lower a chair to get a table height that is right for you. Adjustable computer keyboard holders allow you to type at lap height so your shoulders can relax. Adjustable computer monitor stands, editors' writing desks, and copy stands, like the one made by KayJae, allow you to read with your eyes looking straight ahead so your head is tucked and chin is level. Whether you're typing or writing, mobile arm supports can hold your arms up so your shoulders don't have to.

Driving is often when spasms frequently get fed, since you're usually more focused on what's happening outside the vehicle than what's going on inside your body. You need to get into painless posture as soon as you get behind the wheel. Adjust your seat angle, height, and distance from the pedals. You can buy a thin auto lumbar cushion and use a "butt lift" if you need to. To keep your shoulder and neck muscles relaxed, place your hands at the eight o'clock and four o'clock positions on the wheel. A spinner knob will allow you to turn the wheel easily with one hand. Before you start driving, tuck your head, get your chin level, and adjust the rearview mirror so you can see behind you. If your head or upper body starts to slump forward, you'll no longer be able to see in the rearview mirror—reminding you to sit right.

THE EVERY-INNING STRETCH

In chapter 10 I mentioned that a physical therapist can help you find a few specific stretches you can do throughout the day to turn off your spasms and keep them turned off. For example, if you sit doing desk or computer work, you should take a break every thirty minutes, get into painless posture, and do a few neck, shoulder, or back muscle stretches. Whenever you stretch, stretch only *away* from the side that is tight or hurts. Stretching in the direction of the pain will just shorten the muscles and feed the spasm. And be careful not to twist back and forth at the waist or roll your head around on your neck because moving "feels better." Spasms occur because your muscles are too active, so remember this Post-Polio Precept, which applies to both pain and weakness:

USE ONLY THE MUSCLES YOU NEED.

Whether you're stretching, moving, or just sitting, try to relax muscles you're not using. Try not to clench your fists, your jaw, or face muscles, or to hold your breath. And try not to do the "Polio Shuffle"—constantly tapping a foot, shifting in your seat, or keeping time to the oompah band in your head with a pencil. Also try to be aware of how you're breathing. Most people are "chest breathers," using their chest, neck, and shoulder muscles, instead of the diaphragm and belly, to move air in and out of their lungs. This is especially true of polio survivors who have paralyzed muscles between their ribs or have stomach muscle weakness. To find out if you're a chest breather, put one hand on your belly and the other on your upper chest below your throat, and take a slow, deep breath. If your belly stays flat and your chest rises, you're a chest breather, turning on and shortening your neck and shoulder muscles every time you take a breath. Learning how to belly-breathe is another way to relax your muscles and get rid of neck and shoulder pain.

STAYING OFF THE ROLLER COASTER

There's one big problem with the management techniques I've described: They work and work quickly. Why would that be a big problem? As soon as polio survivors slow down and feel better, they begin the roller coaster. They think their PPS are "cured," revert to their old Type A, use-it-or-lose-it ways, and resume doing all the things that triggered symptoms in the first place. And guess what? The symptoms come right back.

Please don't let this happen to you! If you manage your PPS and stay off the roller coaster, you can expect—without pills and without muscle-strengthening exercises—to feel stronger and function better for years to come. If you don't fully care for yourself and keep using it, you will keep losing it.

It seems that eventually every polio survivor will develop some problem related to having had polio. Sooner or later your remaining poliovirus-damaged, overworked neurons, overstressed muscles, and overloaded joints are going to start complaining—and with good reason. Will every polio survivor eventually develop every PPS symptom, from fatigue to muscle weakness to trouble swallowing? Absolutely not. But all polio survivors, whether they have symptoms right now or not, should follow The Golden Rule and remember this Post-Polio Precept:

A POUND OF PREVENTION IS WORTH A TON OF THERAPY.

The Golden Rule does not mean that polio survivors should sit home and become couch potatoes. It does mean that you should listen to your body and change the way you live so you can manage the symptoms you have and prevent PPS *before* they start.

CHAPTER 17

Fatigue By Any Other Name

Fatigue and weakness are my life. What limits me most is being mentally drained, being unable to focus or think clearly. After mental or physical effort or emotional stress, I feel as though the blood has been drained from my brain. When I overuse my arms I have muscle weakness, which, if I ignore it, can lead to overwhelming fatigue and a dizzy feeling. Any kind of overwork or severe stress will bring on muscle twitching and a profoundly stiff neck. Another problem is the replacement of a previously "cast-iron stomach" with new bothersome gastrointestinal problems. And I also have cold feet.

Luckily time, and an appreciation of the importance of rest and pacing, have led to much greater control of all of my symptoms. When fatigue is prevented, difficulty with focusing, thinking clearly, and remembering also decrease. Learning to slow down, rather than push myself harder, was extraordinarily difficult. There were the internal and external voices I heard daily: "Don't be such a slacker," "Try harder," "Do more," "Get more exercise," and "Get over it." I still have a tendency to overestimate my daily allotment of energy and to take on more than I can do. And the "brick wall" returns on days when I forget to pace myself. But I do feel better.

BETTY, CLASS OF ?

Cincinnati, 1947. The summer arrives bringing heat, humidity . . . and fear. Polio is coming again and the terror has never been greater. The year 1946 had brought America's worst epidemic to date, the death rate rising to an all-time high. But as July became August and then September, there was an eerie calm in Cincinnati. While there had been 167 cases of polio during a previous summer, only forty cases had been reported by the end of August. Why were there so few cases of polio? Had "The Summer Plague" miraculously come to an end? No, the poliovirus had not disappeared. It was attacking Cincinnati at that very moment. It's just that no one recognized its disguise.

For at least four weeks during August and early September, Cincinnati pediatricians saw a new illness they called the Summer Grippe. Its symptoms—fever, headache, stomach pain, nausea, sore throat, and generalized aching—came on suddenly in children between one and ten years old. The kids were not sick enough to go to the hospital and saw their family doctor once if at all. That summer Albert Sabin was listening to his colleagues talking about Summer Grippe. He concluded that there were at least ten thousand cases; in some parts of the city hardly a child escaped.

Why was Sabin, a preeminent polio researcher, interested in the Summer Grippe? Because many of the children had a stiff neck, the red-flag symptom that usually required immediate hospitalization and the terrifying diagnosis: "Poliomyelitis." However, since Summer Grippe did not lead to paralysis and symptoms disappeared within a week, pediatricians were not interested in hospitalizing children. But Sabin was. He remembered the unusual flu that had struck Denmark during August and September 1934; although there were just one hundred cases of polio, and only twenty-seven patients were paralyzed, six hundred more reported a "slight fever." He wondered if some mild form of poliovirus could have caused the 1934 summer flu in Denmark and was causing Summer Grippe in Cincinnati. Sabin decided to find out.

A Medical Detective Story

Sabin admitted thirteen children with Summer Grippe symptoms to The Children's Hospital. The kids had fevers of around 103, almost all were listless and had headaches, many had sore throats, and most had stomach pain. These fluish, feverish, and sometimes fussy children had spinal taps; body fluid specimens were also taken. Eight were diagnosed with Summer Grippe. Two had stiff necks and were diagnosed with "nonparalytic" polio. One child was diagnosed with "dysentery," another "rhinitis," and a third "pneumonia." None of the children was seriously ill, and they all left the hospital in about nine days.

With the children gone, Sabin returned to his laboratory to look for poliovirus in the specimens he had collected. Remarkably, Sabin found antibodies to the Lansing poliovirus in the blood of five of the eight children with Summer Grippe and in one of the two children with "nonparalytic" polio. Sabin then exposed monkeys to the fluids he had collected, watched the animals for about a month to see if weakness or paralysis developed, and ultimately performed autopsies to look for the neuron damage that is the unique calling card of the poliovirus. Fluids from Summer Grippe patients paralyzed one monkey and damaged brain-activating system and spinal cord motor neurons in others.

A Kinder, Gentler Poliovirus?

Sabin concluded that a low-virulence or "mild" Lansing poliovirus caused the flu-like symptoms of the Summer Grippe. Although Sabin's mild poliovirus did not cause muscle weakness—let alone paralysis—in humans, it did something even the most virulent paralytic poliovirus had never done: sicken at least ten thousand kids in the city during one summer. At its worst the virulent paralytic poliovirus felled only 167 Cincinnati residents.

Yet not everyone agreed that a kinder, gentler poliovirus

caused the Summer Grippe, not even the editor of the journal that published Sabin's findings. Enter David Bodian once again, this time as the editor of the *American Journal of Hygiene*. Bodian told Sabin in a letter that the evidence supporting the conclusion that a low-virulence "mild" poliovirus caused the Summer Grippe was "very far from being satisfactory," and that the paper he submitted to Bodian for publication would be "subject to serious criticisms." Bodian had certainly earned the right to criticize Sabin's conclusions, since it was Bodian who'd discovered the significant extent to which even a "nonparalytic" poliovirus could damage the brain stem and spinal cord. But Bodian should have been the one scientist to readily accept Sabin's claim that a mild poliovirus not only caused Summer Grippe symptoms but also killed neurons, although not enough neurons to cause weakness or even a stiff neck. He did not. Bodian wrote Sabin that he had not proved a "causal relationship" between the poliovirus and the Summer Grippe, saying, "it is equally plausible to assume" that the poliovirus "was found in accidental relationship with the illness."

Sabin wrote back, countering that fluid collected during the same period from twenty-four patients with "nonparalytic" polio did not cause nerve damage in monkeys, supporting his claim that he had "caught" a unique poliovirus that both caused Summer Grippe symptoms and damaged neurons in monkeys at a much higher rate than did even the "nonparalytic" poliovirus floating around Cincinnati that summer. But Sabin could not actually prove a causal relationship between his "mild" poliovirus and the Summer Grippe, admitting to Bodian, "It is, in fact [a] matter of probable guilt by association." Sabin was missing important cards if his claims were to trump Bodian's criticisms. One card Sabin wouldn't hold until 1952; the final card wouldn't be dealt until 1955.

In 1947 only one poliovirus—the Lansing type—had been identified and its antibodies measured. As I mentioned in chapter 3, it wasn't until two years later that David Bodian himself found that there were three individual types of poliovirus that caused illness in humans—Brunhilde, Lansing, and Leon, renamed poliovirus Types I, II, and III. In 1952 Sabin tested body fluids saved from his 1947 paralytic and "nonparalytic" polio patients for all three polioviruses. He discovered only Type I antibodies and concluded that a Type I "high-virulence" poliovirus—and not the Type II virus—was responsible for cases of paralytic and "nonparalytic" polio in 1947. So Sabin was right: Type I and Type II polioviruses were circulating simultaneously in Cincinnati that summer. But did a low-virulence Type II virus cause the Summer Grippe and somehow prevent the high-virulence Type I poliovirus from causing "typical polio"? The answer would be found thousands of miles east of Cincinnati.

To Iceland from the Heartland

In September 1948 three cases of paralytic polio were diagnosed in the small city of Akureyri, Iceland. And although not another case of polio was reported, over the next few months more than eleven hundred Icelanders reported typical polio symptoms— fever, neck pain, muscle weakness, and even some paralysis—as well as tingling, numbness, and "general tiredness," symptoms that are not associated with polio. Although fluid samples from four Icelanders were sent to David Bodian's laboratory for testing, neither the poliovirus nor poliovirus antibodies were found. Yet doctors in Iceland concluded that there were only two possible causes for what has come to be known as "Iceland disease": Either a mild strain of poliovirus was responsible for the epidemic, or some unknown neuron-damaging virus had been present.

Hard evidence for a mild strain of poliovirus causing Iceland disease was not available for six more years. In 1955 there was an extensive polio epidemic in Iceland caused by the Type I poliovirus. In addition, there were two new outbreaks of Iceland disease. Remarkably, not one case of polio was reported in towns where there was Iceland disease, despite the fact that only 7 percent of the children tested in those towns had Type I antibodies. Equally remarkable, 100 percent of children tested in the Iceland disease towns had antibodies to Type II poliovirus, as well as high levels of antibodies to the rare Type III poliovirus. Just as Sabin thought happened in Cincinnati, children in Iceland had been exposed to a mild Type II poliovirus that damaged their brains and spinal cords, causing symptoms of Iceland disease— but also preventing infection by the high-virulence Type I paralytic poliovirus.

How could an infection by one poliovirus type prevent infection by another type without benefit of protective antibodies? That answer came during the 1959 Singapore study of Sabin's own oral polio vaccine. Children were given a vaccine that contained all three live but "attenuated" polioviruses—that is, specially grown polioviruses that stimulate antibody production but do not damage neurons. Unexpectedly, the Type II poliovirus was found to be dominant over the other two types. Just as a flock of dominant and aggressive blue jays blocks less aggressive robins from roosting in your backyard, the dominant Type II poliovirus blocks all other polioviruses—even the naturally occurring Type I poliovirus that was causing Singapore's 1959 polio epidemic—from multiplying and latching on to poliovirus receptors. So children in Iceland and Singapore were protected from getting paralytic polio because a mild Type II poliovirus elbowed-out the high-virulent Type I poliovirus.

So Sabin was right again. A mild Type II poliovirus protected the children of Cincinnati from the Type I poliovirus, but at the price of giving them the Summer Grippe. In retrospect this point had already been proved. When the Summer Grippe epidemic reached its peak at the end of August, there had been no more than forty reported cases of polio. Only after the Summer Grippe's Type II poliovirus had left town in mid-September did polio cases start to increase, reaching a total of 170, the highest number in Cincinnati history to date.

Polio By Any Other Name?

Knowing that there have been comparatively mild poliovirus outbreaks that damaged the brain and sometimes the spinal cord without causing paralysis or even weakness may dispose of some long-standing Polio Fictions, explain new findings about PPS, and solve a mystery that's nearly sixty years old.

One Polio Fiction has already been banished: We know that "nonparalytic" polio is a misnomer. David Bodian showed in 1949, and Alan McComas confirmed in 1997, that paralytic and "nonparalytic" polio are not separate conditions but a single disease whose obvious symptoms are determined by the location and number of neurons killed by the poliovirus. Bodian even found that more brain stem neurons can be damaged, and damaged more extensively, in "nonparalytic" than in paralytic polio. As a matter of fact, the location of damaged brain neurons Bodian found in "nonparalytic" polio was the same as in monkeys injected with body fluids from Sabin's Summer Grippe patients. What's more, some people with "nonparalytic" polio have damage only in the brain stem and not in the spinal cord.

The finding that damage to the brain-activating system may be the only damage after poliovirus infection could explain why fatigue is reported more frequently than muscle weakness in both paralytic and "nonparalytic" polio survivors, as well as our Surveys' finding of no relationship between the severity of post-polio fatigue and the number of limbs originally paralyzed or the severity of the polio attack, as indicated by whether polio survivors had been hospitalized or the length of their hospital stay.

What's more, a mystery dating from 1934 may finally be solved by understanding the brain-altering effects of even a "mild" poliovirus. In 1934 an illness resembling Iceland disease struck 150 doctors and nurses who were caring for polio patients at the Los Angeles General Hospital. Since 1934 there have been more than three dozen outbreaks of a similar illness that was at first diagnosed as "poliomyelitis," then as "abortive" or "atypical poliomyelitis," and finally named "myalgic encephalomyelitis," meaning muscle pain with inflammation of the brain and spinal cord. *Myalgic encephalomyelitis,* or *ME,* was coined by British infectious disease specialist Melvin Ramsay when three hundred staff members of London's Royal Free Hospital became ill in 1955 with symptoms identical to those seen in Los Angeles twenty-one years earlier.

As with polio, the initial ME symptoms included headache, neck pain, low-grade fever, and muscle pain, often followed by weakness. ME patients were irritable and anxious, overwhelmingly sleepy, and had brain wave slowing and "conspicuous changes in their levels of concentration" that persisted for months after the acute illness, signs and symptoms common among children who had recovered from polio. But unlike polio, paralysis was very rare, there were frequent reports of numbness or tingling, and there were hardly any breathing problems—and almost invariably no deaths. Also unlike polio, some of the acute symptoms of ME remained for years. Many patients continued to have "exhaustion and fatigability" that were "always made worse by exercise and emotional stress," and had persistent poor concentration, word-finding difficulty, and "an inordinate desire to sleep." Some ME patients reported fatigue, that they were "not as quick or incisive in thought" as before their illness, "a decreased ability to learn, and a decline in their short-term memory" that lasted for decades. Some patients from the 1934 Los Angeles outbreak never recovered.

Despite the differences between polio and ME, an association with the poliovirus was suggested by the fact that of more than a dozen ME outbreaks before the introduction of the polio vaccine in 1954, nine occurred during or immediately after outbreaks of polio, and several involved hospital staff who cared for polio patients.

MORE UNRECOGNIZED EPIDEMICS

Could it be that, as in Cincinnati and in Iceland, a "mild" "nonparalytic" poliovirus was responsible for ME outbreaks? Perhaps. But we'll never know. The few times it was looked for, poliovirus was not found in ME patients. And once the polio vaccine had been distributed, none of the polioviruses could have caused ME in anyone who had been vaccinated.

But something unexpected, frightening, and totally unrecognized happened after the polio vaccine was distributed: The number of ME cases went through the roof. In 1972 Ramsay was joined by another British infectious disease specialist, Elizabeth Dowsett, who inherited all of Ramsay's patients and their records upon his death in 1990. In 1998 Dowsett, founder of the CFS Diagnostic and Management Service in Essex, England, reviewed the twenty-five hundred ME patients she or Ramsay had seen since 1919, and plotted the cases of ME against reported cases of polio. When the Salk and then Sabin vaccines brought the yearly number of British polio cases below twenty-five in the early 1960s, the number of ME patients took off. In Ramsay's and Dowsett's practice alone, between 1960 and 1980 the number of ME patients increased fiftyfold. Between 1980 and 1990, the number of patients with ME increased yet again by a factor of fifty! Throughout the world, thirty-two ME outbreaks were recorded after the polio vaccine was distributed. Something other than the poliovirus was causing ME.

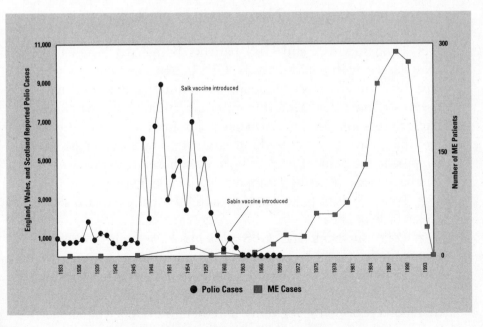

U.K. REPORTED POLIO CASES AND ME PATIENTS

PPS, CFS, and ME Parallels

But while British ME cases skyrocketed unnoticed during the 1980s, a "new" disease discovered in the United States got lots of attention. Residents of Nevada reported strange symptoms—fatigue, difficulty concentrating, and aching muscles—that were called "chronic fatigue syndrome." At first CFS was dismissively nicknamed "yuppie flu." CFS was said to be a psychosomatic disorder, a form of emotional exhaustion or depression, that was thought to give overworked, affluent, upwardly mobile twenty-somethings an acceptable way out of their superstressed work lives. But research since 1984 has compiled more and more evidence that CFS and ME are physical, not emotional, illnesses. What's more, our studies and Surveys, combined with those of other researchers, have found remarkable similarities between the signs and symptoms of post-polio brain fatigue, CFS, and ME:

- Polio survivors and CFS/ME patients report disabling fatigue that is triggered or made worse by physical exertion and emotional stress.
- Polio survivors and CFS patients both have "overactive" lifestyles. As with polio survivors, CFS patients are worriers who have very stressful, overextended, overcommitted lives that leave them straining for achievement, perfection, and constantly feeling pressured for time. Also like polio survivors, CFS patients feel they "have to do everything" and try to make other people happy—to the point of neglecting or even harming themselves—and have great difficulty disappointing people by saying no.
- Nearly half of polio survivors and CFS patients have sleep apnea or hypopneas.
- Polio survivors and CFS patients have belly problems, including decreased contraction of the intestines.
- In polio survivors and CFS patients there is a relationship between fainting and fatigue. In both groups purple feet indicate that blood pools in the leg veins, and there is evidence of damage to the nerves that control skin blood vessels.

• Polio survivors with fatigue and CFS/ME patients report difficulty with attention, word finding, thinking quickly, and memory. On neuropsychologic testing, attention and word finding are abnormal and thinking ability is slowed in fatigued polio survivors and CFS patients. Despite these difficulties, both groups of patients have high-normal or above-normal IQs and have no impairments of memory or thinking. Both groups have been found to have more years of education and are more likely to be professionals than the general population.

• Up to 85 percent of patients with CFS have brain wave slowing similar to that seen immediately after polio and which we have found in fatigued polio survivors.

• White spots were found on MRI in the brain's myelinated neurons in fatigued polio survivors and in CFS patients. These white spots are similar to but smaller than those in the brains of multiple sclerosis patients, who also can have severe fatigue and difficulty focusing attention.

• White spots were found on MRIs in the gray neurons of the brain-activating system in polio survivors with fatigue and in one study of CFS patients. The SPECT scanner, a newer brain-imaging device that has not yet been used to study polio survivors, has found decreased activity of brain stem neurons in two studies of CFS patients.

• Fatigued polio survivors and CFS patients release less of the brain-activating hormone ACTH.

• More prolactin is released in fatigued polio survivors and CFS patients, suggesting that less of the brain-activating neurochemical dopamine is being produced in both groups. U.S. veterans diagnosed with Gulf War syndrome, who report symptoms similar to those in polio survivors with brain fatigue and CFS patients, were found to have less brain dopamine in the basal ganglia and abnormalities of brain stem neurons that are part of the brain-activating system.

• Growth hormone is lower in polio survivors with new muscle weakness and in CFS patients. Since growth hormone release is stimulated by dopamine, it's possible that damage to brain dopamine neurons causes lower growth hormone levels in polio survivors and CFS patients. Since there was no improvement when growth hormone was given to polio survivors or CFS patients, lower growth hormone levels are most likely the result of damage to the brain and not the direct cause of fatigue or muscle weakness.

DOES THE POLIOVIRUS CAUSE CFS?

The striking parallels between the signs, symptoms, and studies of post-polio fatigue, ME, and CFS caused us to propose the Brain Fatigue Generator model of post-viral fatigue syndromes. The Brain Fatigue Generator model says that it's normal for neurons in the brain stem and basal ganglia to become "tired" during the course of the day. This tiredness decreases brain activation and produces typical feelings of fatigue: difficulty paying attention, not wanting to get out of a chair, and the overwhelming desire to just slip between the sheets and go to sleep. After a good night's sleep in those who don't have PPS or CFS/ME, brain-activating system neurons are refreshed, and fatigue disappears. However, in PPS, ME and CFS patients, fatigue is not relieved by sleep, because brain-activating neurons were damaged and are never refreshed. The symptoms of fatigue—in both polio survivors and CFS/ME patients—result from a virus damaging brain-activating neurons.

The CFS research community was excited by the Brain Fatigue Generator model because it explained post-polio fatigue for which there is a complete chain of evidence: We know which virus damaged brain-activating neurons, and we have MRI, EEG, hormonal—even autopsy evidence—of that damage, which is related to the signs and symptoms of fatigue. In 1995 we were asked to present the BFG model at the First World Congress on Chronic Fatigue Syndrome in Brussels, on which CFS specialist David Bell commented in *The CFIDS Chronicle*:

What seems extraordinary is the similarity of the

residual deficits caused by poliovirus and the clinical
symptoms present in chronic fatigue syndrome. The similarities are tantalizing. For years we have been looking for
an anatomic model of chronic fatigue, particularly post-
infectious fatigue. Is it possible that the post-polio syndrome is an example of CFS caused by a specific infectious
agent? The work by Dr. Bruno and co-workers may become
immensely important not only to the many persons who
suffered polio but to those with CFS as well.

Given the "tantalizing" similarities, could CFS and ME be
caused today by a "mild" poliovirus infection? Absolutely not. As
we discussed, anyone vaccinated against polio would be immune
to all polioviruses, including those that caused the Summer
Grippe, Iceland disease, and that might have been responsible
for ME in the years before the vaccine.

But there may very well be a link between polio, the skyrock-
eting of ME cases in Britain, and the appearance of CFS in the
United States. It may be that the vaccine that eliminated polio
had an unintended consequence. The elimination of poliovirus
left a vacuum that had to be filled. It was the blue jays versus the
robins again. But this time the blue jays were all three
polioviruses and the robins were other members of the
enterovirus family to which polioviruses belong. Apparently all
three polioviruses had been blue jays, dominant over the other
enteroviruses in their ability to multiply in the intestines. With
poliovirus disappearing in vaccinated countries, other
enteroviruses took over the polioviruses' intestinal breeding
ground and filled the vacuum. With polioviruses gone, other
enteroviruses were able to multiply, spill into the bloodstream,
and enter the brain.

In 1990 Elizabeth Dowsett looked for antibodies to nonpolio
enteroviruses in her ME patients. Fifty percent had antibodies to
the first nonpolio enterovirus ever discovered, the Coxsackie B
virus, named for Coxsackie, New York, the town where it was
found to have paralyzed children in 1948. Yes, paralyzed. It isn't
just the polioviruses that enter and kill neurons in the spinal cord

and brain-activating system. Neuron damage, weakness, paralysis, and symptoms of brain fatigue caused by enteroviruses can be so similar to that caused by polioviruses as to be indistinguishable. One Coxsackie virus, named A7, produces paralytic symptoms so similar to polio that it has been named poliovirus Type IV. Other nonpolio enteroviruses that cause damage and symptoms similar to the polioviruses include all the other Coxsackie viruses, the ECHO viruses (which in 1956 were the first viruses associated with an ME outbreak), enterovirus 71, and viruses that cause illnesses that evoke some faraway places with strange-sounding names: central European encephalomyelitis, Australian X, Japanese B, and St. Louis encephalitis. The only direct evidence linking an enterovirus, damage to the brain-activating system, and CFS came in 1994. A thirty-two-year-old woman who had had CFS for five years took her own life. Her autopsy revealed Coxsackie B virus—the same virus for which Dowsett found antibodies in her patients—in both the hypothalamus and brain stem, the very heart of the brain-activating system.

Remembrance of Children Past

On the way back from the 1995 CFS conference in Brussels, we stopped in London and met Elizabeth Dowsett for the first time. She described her experience with ME, not only in adults but also in children. Despite my knowing about the Summer Grippe and Iceland disease, it had never occurred to me that children were getting ME today. Dowsett's experience with children echoed a familiar and disturbing past.

In 1988 Dowsett studied an outbreak of what she calls "Summer Flu" in British grade school students in East Anglia. A quarter of the children in the school district had the flu that summer, and about 10 percent remained ill when school began in the fall. The children reported "profound fatigue and difficulty with memory, attention and were falling asleep during the day"— symptoms that had not improved when children were contacted two years later. Because of this outbreak of what she thought was

ME, Dowsett decided to study a much larger group of school-children to see just how common chronic fatigue was in children after they'd had what appeared to be the flu.

In 1995 she sent questionnaires to nearly three thousand British schools and surveyed 330,000 children. She found that nearly 10 percent had had an illness that looked like ME. Half were unable to go to school and had to be tutored at home; the rest required modified class schedules because of difficulty with focusing attention, thinking clearly, word finding, and staying awake during the day. These symptoms reminded us of the students with Iceland disease and Edith Meyer's description of kids who returned to school after having had polio, whom she found to have "fatigability and fleeting attention."

The parallels between Elizabeth Dowsett's findings in children with chronic fatigue, young people with Iceland disease, and polio survivors were too great to be ignored. When we returned to the United States, I applied to the CFIDS Association of America and received a grant to perform the first study of brain functioning in young people with CFS. We studied a baker's dozen subjects who met the 1994 Centers for Disease Control criteria for CFS, were on average sixteen years old, and had no psychological diagnoses. We compared these CFS kids to ten nonfatigued young people. We found that the more fatigue CFS kids reported, the more difficulty they had staying awake during the day, concentrating, and focusing attention. We administered all the tests of attention, concentration, thinking, and memory that we have used since 1992 to study fatigue in polio survivors. As we have found in adult polio survivors with fatigue, as others have found in adults with CFS, and as Edith Meyer found in young people who had polio, attention test scores were either abnormal or significantly lower in the fatigued kids than in those without CFS.

With this study the circle had been completed. Individuals with chronic fatigue—be they adults or young people, polio survivors, those with CFS or ME—share an inability to stay awake during the day, to concentrate, and to focus attention. We think the simplest explanation for these findings is the Brain Fatigue

Generator model: that various viruses damage the brain-activating system, damage that causes the signs and symptoms of chronic fatigue.

Baby Boom Bust

Elizabeth Dowsett believes that a nonpolio enterovirus, most likely a Coxsackie virus, is causing CFS and ME in those born since the polio vaccine. But there is another scenario you may find surprising, or that may already have occurred to you. In a survey of nearly twenty thousand Americans, researcher Leonard Jason found that half of everyone with CFS is over forty years old. He concluded that baby boomers may in fact be at greater risk for CFS.

Forty-plus baby boomers at greater risk for CFS? Why does this ring a bell? Remember that, although the polio vaccine was developed in 1954, it took until 1959 for there to be fewer than ten thousand cases of polio each year in the United States. So anyone born before 1960 was at risk for getting polio. Those who were not vaccinated, who did have polio, and are reporting fatigue today are being diagnosed with PPS. But what about the estimated 160,000 Americans who had "nonparalytic" polio before the vaccine was developed but were never diagnosed? And what of the untold tens of thousands who had Summer Grippe? According to Lenny Jason's calculations, potentially half the people who have CFS today may have had an undiagnosed polio infection when they were children, in the years before the polio vaccine became available, and have brain-activating system damage that is causing their chronic fatigue symptoms today. Could it be that as many as half of everyone diagnosed with chronic fatigue syndrome actually had polio and have PPS, *not* CFS?

To find out, we went back to Cincinnati. In 1999, with the help of the *Cincinnati Post* newspaper and a local television station, the story of the Summer Grippe was told. We asked for anyone who had had Summer Grippe, and especially any of

Sabin's kids—those whom he admitted to Children's Hospital in 1947—to contact us. Despite Albert Sabin's calculation that at least ten thousand children had had Summer Grippe, we received only a dozen letters and phone calls, and not one from someone Sabin had hospitalized. The mild symptoms of Summer Grippe were apparently far from memorable. So we cast the net much more widely.

We developed a questionnaire and, with the help of Elizabeth Dowsett in the United Kingdom and Lydia Nelson and Canada's National ME/FM Action Network, conducted the 2001 International Chronic Fatigue Survey. We asked Americans, Britons, and Canadians with CFS or ME if they'd had a childhood illness—a fever that left them fatigued for several days, maybe a stiff neck, or even muscle weakness—in the years before the polio vaccine was distributed in 1955. Two-thirds of the 586 chronic fatigue patients who responded were born before 1955; they were on average sixty-one years old, just four years younger than polio survivors' average age in our Surveys, which again dashed the notion of chronic fatigue syndrome being a "yuppie flu." Symptoms of brain fatigue were more frequent and more severe in all chronic fatigue patients than they were among the polio survivors we have surveyed. Physical stress triggered symptoms in more than 90 percent of both the 2001 Survey's chronic fatigue patients and polio survivors in our 1985 Survey. More than 90 percent of chronic fatigue patients surveyed reported that emotional stress triggered symptoms as compared to almost 60 percent of polio survivors in the 1985 Survey. While nearly three-quarters of polio survivors in our Surveys were women, 90 percent of chronic fatigue patients surveyed were female, a percentage nearly identical to the number of women affected in the 1948 Iceland disease outbreak.

Twenty percent of surveyed chronic fatigue patients born before 1955 remembered having had an illness with a fever, typically at age seven in 1947, the same year as Cincinnati's Summer Grippe epidemic. Just over one-third recalled having had a stiff neck—the red-flag symptom of a virus infecting the brain and spinal cord—about one-third were hospitalized, and

70 percent remember having had muscle weakness. The distribution of childhood illness cases in the Survey is nearly identical to the distribution of reported polio cases in the United States and United Kingdom between 1935 and 1955:

	1935–1940	1941–1945	1946–1950	1951–1955
Polio cases	8%	12%	28%	44%
Childhood illness	5%	12%	30%	46%

Chronic fatigue patients who remember having had a childhood illness before 1955 were different from both those without a childhood illness and from polio survivors. Difficulty with concentration, thinking clearly, word finding, and joint pain were reported to be about 15 percent more frequent in chronic fatigue patients who'd had a childhood illness than among those without. Nearly 80 percent of childhood illness patients reported that cold triggered their symptoms, versus nearly 70 percent of chronic fatigue patients without a childhood illness and 60 percent of the polio survivors we surveyed in 1985. Chronic fatigue patients without a childhood illness and all of the polio survivors we've surveyed had the same average Type A score of fifty-five, while childhood illness patients scored sixty-four.

While just over 60 percent of polio survivors in our 1985 Survey reported muscle twitching at night, almost three-quarters of chronic fatigue patients without a childhood illness reported nighttime twitching, as compared to 95 percent of childhood illness patients. Symptoms of abnormal breathing during sleep—snoring, waking short of breath or with heart pounding—were reported by half of chronic fatigue patients without a childhood illness and by almost two-thirds of childhood illness patients. As we've discussed, about 50 percent of our PPS patients had abnormal breathing during sleep.

Childhood illness patients reported they had fainted seven times on average since they have had chronic fatigue, while polio survivors responding to our 1995 Survey reported fainting an average of only two times during their lifetime, as did chronic fatigue patients without a childhood illness. However, just as in polio survivors, neither being hospitalized nor having muscle weakness associated with the childhood illness were related to brain fatigue symptoms today.

The findings of the 2001 Chronic Fatigue Survey support the notion that a mild childhood illness occurring before polio vaccination began in 1955—possibly resulting from the Type II poliovirus responsible for Summer Grippe and Iceland disease or a Type I poliovirus causing "nonparalytic" polio—damaged reticular formation neurons and the brain-activating system, setting the stage for midlife symptoms that are identical to post-polio brain fatigue. In almost every way, chronic fatigue patients who remember having had a childhood illness are more like polio survivors with brain fatigue than are post-polio patients themselves: They actually have more difficulty with brain fatigue symptoms, are more Type A and more affected by emotional stress, have had more episodes of fainting, and are more likely to have sleep disturbed by abnormal breathing and muscle twitching. So when baby boomers report symptoms of chronic fatigue, doctors need to ask if there is a history of childhood illness with a fever—and maybe a stiff neck or muscle weakness—that occurred during the polio epidemic years, even though it may be relatively rare for patients to remember such a mild illness. But whether or not chronically fatigued patients recall a childhood illness, the findings that more than 50 percent of all of those surveyed had symptoms of abnormal nighttime breathing and that 80 percent had nighttime muscle twitching requires that a sleep history be taken as in polio survivors—from both patients and their bed partners—and that sleep studies be performed so that disturbed sleep can be ruled out or treated as a cause of chronic fatigue.

A Final Tender Point

It is disturbing to think that, as an unintended consequence of polio vaccination, enteroviruses have filled the vacuum left by the polioviruses. Even more disturbing is that doctors choose to ignore more than eighty years of research indicating that ME, and its American cousin CFS, are very likely caused by one or more of the enteroviruses. More than polio survivors with PPS, those with ME and CFS have been dismissed as lazy, crazy, or outright liars by the medical community. Maybe it's our Puritan heritage, but there are two symptoms by which people are not "allowed" to be disabled: fatigue and pain. Unfortunately, there is yet another condition, characterized by chronic pain and linked to CFS, that doctors refuse to believe has a physical basis.

Fibromyalgia is a syndrome of muscle and joint pain that is defined by areas of tenderness to touch, called "tender points," in specific locations: over the buttocks, upper chest, knees, and elbows, as well as in the hip, back, shoulder, and neck muscles. Because fibromyalgia patients can have chronic fatigue, and because CFS patients can have muscle pain, some doctors believe that CFS and fibromyalgia are the same condition, even though not all CFS patients have pain and not all fibromyalgia patients have fatigue. Still, the similarities between fibromyalgia and CFS are remarkable, as are the parallels between fibromyalgia and PPS:

• Polio survivors report joint, muscle, neck, and back pain at least as frequently as do those with fibromyalgia.
• The neurochemical enkephalin, the body's own morphine, is decreased in fibromyalgia patients. We've discussed that neurons in both the brain and spinal cord that produce enkephalin were killed by the poliovirus. Lower amounts of enkephalin may explain both fibromyalgia patients' increased sensitivity to touch at tender points and our finding of polio survivors' doubled sensitivity to pain.
• Growth hormone is lower in polio survivors reporting new

muscle weakness and in those with fibromyalgia, as it is in CFS patients. Administering growth hormone decreased pain in one study of fibromyalgia patients, but had no beneficial effect when given to polio survivors or CFS patients.

• More prolactin is released in fibromyalgia patients, as it is in CFS patients and in polio survivors with fatigue.

• Fibromyalgia patients have decreased activity in basal ganglia, thalamus, and brain stem neurons, parts of the brain-activating system damaged by the poliovirus and whose activity is also decreased in CFS patients.

• Fibromyalgia patients require more time to successfully complete attention tests, as do CFS patients and polio survivors with fatigue.

• Like polio survivors, fibromyalgia patients have a decreased ability to make blood vessels constrict, suggesting that they have damage to sympathetic nerves that control the veins, as do polio survivors.

• Sleep apnea is seen in nearly half of those with fibromyalgia and in nearly half of our post-polio patients.

• At least one-third of adults and children with fibromyalgia have sleep that is disturbed by involuntary leg movements like those seen in polio survivors.

Given the overlap of symptoms in fibromyalgia and CFS, nonpolio enteroviruses might cause both conditions by damaging the same neurons that were attacked by the polioviruses, damage we think is responsible for the symptoms of PPS. Indeed, antibodies to our old enterovirus friend Coxsackie B virus, as well as Pogosta and hepatitis C enteroviruses, have been found in fibromyalgia patients. And it may also be possible that baby boomers are misdiagnosed with fibromyalgia, as they may be misdiagnosed with CFS, when in fact they had an undiagnosed case of polio in childhood and now have PPS.

The New Polio

In September 2002, for the first time the mosquito-borne West Nile virus was reported to be causing "polio-like paralysis"—in arms, legs and even breathing muscles—placing several people on respirators.

Polio, paralysis and respirators. These words strike fear not only in the nearly two million North Americans alive today who had polio, but also in those who lived through the polio epidemics that terrorized the world fifty years ago. Despite there being only a handful of West Nile paralytic "polio" cases so far, it is frightening that the symptoms of and damage done to the brain and spinal cord by the West Nile and polioviruses—different viruses transmitted in different ways—are so similar.

- Nearly 1 percent of those infected with WNV have paralysis, almost the same percentage as in those infected with polioviruses;
- Up to 15 percent of those severely affected with West Nile encephalitis die, while about 15 percent of all "bulbar" polio patients died due to severe brain stem encephalitis;
- The West Nile virus may be mutating and becoming more virulent since it is now paralyzing younger individuals, just as the poliovirus did in the 1950s.

There was another first in 2002. New Yorkers admitted to hospital with West Nile encephalitis in 1999 were reported to have lasting symptoms: two-thirds have chronic fatigue, half reported difficulty with walking and memory, 44 percent have muscle weakness, and more than one-third are depressed. Said New York City assistant health commissioner Marcelle Layton, "Many people don't realize that [West Nile] is not an infection that you always get over."

Except for depression, the percentage of West Nile encephalitis patients reporting chronic symptoms is lower than polio survivors with PPS. Yet, despite the increasing similarities between West Nile patients and polio survivors, in terms of acute and chronic symptoms as well as brain and spinal cord damage, those who had West Nile virus are "believed" when thay complain of lasting fatigue and muscle weakness—and even depression—while doctors still don't "believe" PPS exists. David Bodian's scores of autopsies performed in the 1940s showed that the encephalitis caused by the poliovirus was far more common and severe than is West Nile encephalitis. So if West Nile encephalitis is accepted as a cause of chronic fatigue, memory loss, and depression, why do doctors think it impossible that poliovirus encephalitis can produce the debilitating fatigue that is the most common PPS symptom? If West Nile virus "is not an infection that you always get over," why do doctors refuse to even consider that other more common encephalitis-causing agents—especially poliovirus cousins such as the Coxsackie viruses—might be responsible for fatigue and memory loss you don't always get over in those with Chronic Fatigue Syndrome?

And what will happen to the reported 20 percent of West Nile patients who have "only a mild case of the flu" and are never diagnosed? As we discussed earlier on, 22 percent of those infected with the poliovirus only had flu-like symptoms, often don't know that they had polio or were diagnosed with "non-paralytic" polio, and are reporting PPS today. Thirty years from now, will undiagnosed West Nile patients who report fatigue and weakness—and even those diagnosed with West Nile virus— find themselves in the same situation as polio survivors and CFS patients, disbelieved and told that they are malingering or that symptoms are all in their heads?

Let's hope that cases of West Nile "polio" will remind doctors that many different viruses can permanently damage the brain and spinal cord and cause lasting symptoms, including fatigue, memory loss and muscle weakness. Let us hope that acceptance of PPS and CFS as post-encephalitic syndrome will prevent West Nile patients from being disbelieved and dismissed if they develop "Post-West Nile Syndrome" three decades from now.

No More Time to Waste

Just like polio survivors, those with CFS, ME, and fibromyalgia have no more time to waste with doctors who don't believe their conditions are real and who think pain and fatigue are "all in their heads." It's time doctors start looking at the cause of chronic fatigue and pain from the brain up, instead of from the mind down, so that adults and young people with chronic fatigue and fibromyalgia start getting help for their symptoms, instead of being blamed for them.

If you have CFS, ME, or fibromyalgia and can't find a doctor to believe you, or can't get to a specialist, you can take treatment into your own hands and start managing your symptoms right now. Ask your local doctor for blood tests to rule out other conditions, especially anemia and a slow thyroid, and have your blood pressure taken lying, sitting, and standing. Ask to have a sleep study. Then start practicing energy conservation, work simplification, taking frequent rest breaks, pacing activities, and living by The Golden Rule. Will these PPS management techniques work for CFS, ME, and fibromyalgia? Melvin Ramsay himself said, "The basic fundamental tenet of the management of a case of ME is REST with graduated activity well within the limitations which the disease imposes." A British survey of more than two thousand people with ME found that pacing reduced symptoms in over 80 percent, while exercise increased symptoms in 50 percent. And, wrote Elizabeth Dowsett:

> There is very little, if any, difference between ME, CFS and PPS. In 1986, I started reading Dr. Bruno's articles on PPS and have used them as guidelines for the management of ME patients ever since. Your programme has amply proved its worth as some 300 Christmas cards from patients all over the UK and from around the world testify. I also have many letters from doctors who say that their patients have truly benefited.

Now is the time for everyone with chronic fatigue or chronic pain from *any* cause to take treatment into their own hands and come to the aid of their bodies. There *is* no more time to waste.

CHAPTER 18

No More Time to Waste

I wasted a year of my life. All of those doctors, those blood tests, needles, and X rays. First the doctors said I was depressed, then they said I needed surgery. They frightened me for no reason and did nothing to help. I could walk by myself when this started. Then I needed a cane, then the walker, and now I'm using a power wheelchair. Because they didn't know what they were doing my legs got worse. I told all of them I had polio and no one listened. What will it take to make them listen?

PATTY, CLASS OF '53

After evaluating, treating, surveying, and studying nearly four thousand polio survivors, what do we know about "post-polio syndrome"? We know that there isn't a specific and consistent group of symptoms that can be considered a syndrome. Polio survivors can have one or any combination of symptoms that can eat away at your ability to function and quality of life; post-polio sequelae—the sequel to having had polio—David Bodian called them. We know that PPS are not caused by the poliovirus or "a polio-like virus" but by the failure of remaining, poliovirus-damaged, overworked brain stem and spinal cord motor neurons, as well as the overuse-abuse of muscles and joints. We know that those who had either paralytic or "nonparalytic" polio can get PPS, and that possibly hundreds of thousands of postwar baby boomers may have had polio and now have PPS in the guise of chronic fatigue syndrome, myalgic encephalomyelitis, or fibromyalgia—even though they are unaware they'd ever *had* polio. And we know that polio survivors can feel better and stay well—maybe even prevent PPS—if they can get their frightened, Type A heads to listen to their tired, pained bodies, decrease physical and emotional stress, and care for themselves maybe for the first time in their lives.

But even in this, the third millennium of PPS, there is one thing we still don't understand: why doctors and governments throughout the world refuse to acknowledge, let alone learn about and provide treatment for PPS. If polio survivors are the best and the brightest, superachievers contributing mightily to society, is it not in every country's best interest to at least keep polio survivors working and paying taxes, to remove the threat of their becoming disabled, unable to work, and going on the dole?

Threats, Both Foreign and Domestic

The American Experience

Fortunately for Americans, the U.S. government does acknowledge the reality of PPS. Medicare pays for PPS treatment. After years of fighting the system, a fight that continues today, the Social Security Administration allows polio survivors who can no longer work to receive disability income. Still, despite twenty years of research on PPS, despite articles published in all the major medical journals, many American doctors—especially neurologists and orthopedists—refuse to believe PPS are real. And since HMOs restrict polio survivors' ability to go out of network to see specialists who are knowledgeable about PPS, treatment options are often severely limited.

But even if referral to a PPS specialist is permitted, services for polio survivors in the United States are dwindling. Only twenty-two states have polio clinics, and nearly two-thirds of the clinics are along the East Coast. Unfortunately, PPS specialists come and go. Of the fourteen U.S. PPS experts who participated in a 1984 conference on PPS, only nine continue to operate PPS centers and treat new patients. In 2001 alone, two U.S. PPS clinics closed and three PPS specialists stopped seeing patients. And it's unlikely new doctors will take up the torch. In the words of one totally uninformed doctor: "It is not profitable to treat polio survivors since the few that are left are in their eighties and are going to die soon anyway."

If the profit motive is limiting services for polio survivors in the United States, you might expect treatment would be more available in countries with socialized medicine. Some countries, such as Norway, Sweden, and Denmark, have had excellent PPS research and treatment centers for decades. But in other countries medicine is anything but socialized when it comes to PPS.

NORTHERN EXPOSURE

In Canada, polio survivors can pick their own general practitioner, but cannot choose their own specialists, such as a physiatrist who knows about PPS. Many general practitioners have never heard of PPS or do not believe PPS is real, so polio survivors are forced to play "doctor roulette," going from GP to GP until they find one who is informed about PPS and willing to refer to a specialist. Yet many specialists are also uninformed about PPS, so referral does not ensure treatment. With the help of an enlightened GP, polio survivors in some parts of Canada can receive outstanding care for PPS. There are several Canadian PPS research and treatment centers. However, even their existence is in jeopardy because the Canadian health system has

another problem: It's broke. Too many people are in need of
health care, and there is not enough tax revenue to pay for it.
Deep federal budget cuts required one PPS clinic to eliminate
its physical therapist until patients mailed in contributions to
pay the therapist's salary. In 2001 the PPS Clinic in Alberta
closed for lack of funding. But the situation is even worse across
"the Pond."

Rue Britannia

I imagined England would be more hospitable to polio survivors,
since a national polio organization has existed there for more
than forty years. But Britain's National Health Service is even
less helpful to polio survivors than is the Canadian system.

Only one hospital is known for treating polio survivors, a
center in London that treated "bulbar" polio in the 1950s. Polio
survivors outside of London need a referral to be treated at that
hospital or at any hospital outside their region. A polio survivor
who was permitted to travel to the hospital was told she should
have "respiratory testing"; nothing was said about her progressive
leg weakness and loss of mobility, let alone having therapy. But
even if that London hospital had provided comprehensive treatment for PPS, how could a single hospital treat all of the estimated 350,000 polio survivors in England, Scotland, and Wales?
The question is now moot, since funding for the hospital's polio
unit has been stopped. A polio clinic is operating in Dublin, but
there is a two-year wait for an evaluation.

Several years ago, polio survivors in the British Midlands
formed polio networks dedicated to providing information and
lobbying local health authorities for comprehensive PPS treatment by local doctors. In 2001 members of the Lincolnshire
Polio Network joined with patients having nervous system diseases—including ME, Guillain-Barre syndrome, multiple sclerosis, Parkinson's disease, and spina bifida—in the Neurological
Alliance. The goal of the alliance is to lobby the NHS to recog-

nize and provide quality care in local communities for everyone who has a neurological illness, including those with PPS and ME. Following their lead, The International Post-Polio Task Force is organizing NAFTA—the North Atlantic Fair Treatment Alliance—to join the approximately five million American, Canadian, and European polio survivors, CFS, and ME patients to lobby governments for benefits and services. The impact of NAFTA was first felt in November 2001 when the health ministers of the European Union agreed to take up the issue of PPS treatment and disability payments for polio survivors at their 2002 meeting.

Fortunately, polio survivors fare better in other Commonwealth countries. There are support networks in Australia and New Zealand in addition to at least a few post-polio clinics.

CONTINENTAL DIVIDE

Once you cross the channel to the Continent, more resources are available for polio survivors. Thriving polio survivor organizations and at least one knowledgeable doctor can be found in Belgium, the Netherlands, Germany, Switzerland, France, the Czech Republic, and Portugal. But the situation worsens again as you move farther south and east. Three polio survivors have had to travel to The Post-Polio Institute from Turkey, where there is no polio survivor organization and no doctor knowledgeable about PPS.

Moving east and south treatment for polio is still inadequate—let alone treatment for PPS—for example, in Pakistan and India. In the Middle East resources exist but are limited. Lebanon has a very dynamic post-polio support group, but Israel has only one doctor knowledgeable about PPS. In the Far East no resources for polio survivors are available in mainland China or in Thailand, although there are polio organizations in Taiwan, Japan, with a group just starting in the Philippines.

Southern Discomfort

In Africa a lone voice has been providing information for polio survivors. Cilla Webster founded The Post-Polio Network SA in 1997. She has funded a newsletter, Internet, and telephone outreach to all Africans through her small pension and dues of $5 U.S. Zimbabwean and Zambian polio survivors are sent the newsletter free of charge because they can't afford membership dues and rely totally on the newsletter for PPS information, since there are no medical personnel knowledgeable about PPS in their countries.

Africa is the primary focus of the polio vaccination effort, where polio was supposed to have been eradicated by the year 2000. In 2000 a conference was held at the United Nations, bringing together third world nations, the World Health Organization, and Rotary International as they recommitted themselves to polio eradication by 2005. Later that year the occurrence of nearly two dozen cases of polio in the Dominican Republic and Haiti, caused by a mutated Type I strain of the oral polio vaccine infecting either unvaccinated or inadequately vaccinated young children, underscored the need for ongoing and complete vaccination.

But who was missing from the table at the UN conference on polio? The world's twenty million polio survivors, those "embarrassing emblems of their own poor timing," as Jane Smith wrote, "clumsy enough to get polio before the vaccine that could have protected them was found." When CNN asked me to comment on the air about the UN conference, I said that it was crucial that all children be vaccinated and that polio be eradicated. But I also said:

> . . . We can't make the same mistake now that we made in 1954, where all of our resources and attention go for the polio vaccine when there are polio survivors now who have PPS, doctors aren't interested, and there are so few resources in the United States and around the world. We have a patient at The Post-Polio Institute right now who

has flown in from Beijing for treatment. We treat people from South Africa, South America, Europe. People from other countries still don't know about PPS and their doctors don't know about PPS.

Unfortunately, the world *is* making the same mistake today that it made in 1954. But it need not. There are sufficient funds and sufficient medical resources to both eradicate polio *and* treat PPS. Unfortunately, polio survivors are no longer adorably pitiful March of Dimes poster children. And although polio survivors are competent, productive adults, they need help now as much as they did forty-eight years ago. Polio vaccination and the treatment of PPS need not be an either–or proposition.

But there is no more time to waste! Please go to the end of this chapter and make copies of The Post-Polio Letter. Mail the letter to each of your doctors and to your government officials, and ask each of your friends—polio survivors or not—to do the same. Let everyone know that polio survivors may be forgotten but are far from gone! Demand the medical services you need to keep working and to maintain your quality of life, and the disability benefits you have earned and deserve.

A Post-Every-Disability Syndrome?

Since PPS reared its frightening head, it has become apparent that late-onset sequelae aren't just for polio survivors anymore. The lessons of PPS being learned by the world's twenty million polio survivors apply to at least another twenty million people throughout the world, since it turns out that anyone who had an early-onset physical disability can develop symptoms identical to PPS:

I was hospitalized and my left leg and right foot were affected. The left leg was reduced in girth and was weak. I made what I thought was a complete recovery and lived a very active life with skiing, jogging, and step aerobics a part

of my daily activities. All that changed about six years ago.
When I did any kind of exercise, about two hours later I
had a cascade of pain moving up my body, starting with the
legs. I now have trouble getting around because my thigh
muscles seem reluctant to do their job. In the last year I
have had to navigate with the help of two canes. In addition the left leg has a propensity to puff up as the day pro-
gresses and I am intolerant to cold.

A weak and atrophied left leg and foot. A complete recovery and
an active life, followed by pain after exercise, then weakened
thigh muscles, needing canes, leg swelling, and cold intolerance.
Sound like polio and PPS? You bet. But Ray's initial illness
occurred in Massachusetts in 1976 after being vaccinated for
the swine flu. Ray didn't have polio; he had Guillain-Barré syndrome. GBS is caused by the immune system attacking not the
neurons but the axons and the myelin insulation surrounding
them. GBS can be triggered by infection with a variety of viruses
(except the poliovirus) and by bacteria. GBS patients have
muscle weakness, breathing difficulty, and difficulty controlling
blood pressure, just as polio patients did. And, as happened following polio, maximum muscle strength returns within about
two years. But unlike polio, GBS damages both motor and sensory neurons, often causing tingling and numbness.

As Ray's story indicates, GBS survivors are developing late-
onset symptoms identical to PPS, including muscle weakness
and cold intolerance, possibly due to the failure of remaining
damaged motor neurons. These new symptoms suggest that the
approximately one million survivors of GBS adopt the "conserve
to preserve" strategy and follow polio survivors' The Golden Rule.

I have never walked without two canes. When I was
thirty-nine I developed nagging left leg pain and weakness
that was diagnosed first as bursitis then sciatica. I could no
longer lift up my right foot so I got a short leg brace. But
the canes have beaten up my shoulders to the point where
I had trouble walking any distance. I had to get a wheel-

chair. But I found that I couldn't push the thing so I had to get a scooter. Even with the scooter, I am feeling more and more fatigued.

Trouble walking any distance, couldn't lift the right foot, got a short leg brace, a wheelchair, then a scooter, plus more and more fatigue. This must be PPS. But it's not. Sara has cerebral palsy, as do about twelve million other people throughout the world. Surveys in the United States, the United Kingdom, and Australia show that those with CP are having the same problems as polio survivors: fatigue, muscle weakness, and pain causing decreased ability to get around, work, and socialize, accompanied by a dose of anxiety and depression.

Just like polio survivors, folk with CP often think their increased symptoms and loss of abilities are the normal effect of getting older; many are told that arthritis is the cause of all their problems. However, as in polio survivors, leg pain is much more likely related to overuse-abuse, and fatigue the result of the increased energy required to haul around a body that is hurting and getting weaker.

Like polio survivors, people with CP develop back and neck pain as muscle weakness causes the head and body to bend forward and to the side. Also like polio survivors, those with CP spent years perfecting their ability to balance and walk with few if any assistive devices, and are loath to "give in" to using braces, canes, crutches, walkers, scooters, or wheelchairs until it becomes "absolutely necessary."

Even though there is no evidence that failing neurons in those with CP cause new weakness, preventing or stopping overuse abuse is the way to manage midlife symptoms.

I had four surgeries before I was seven and I have always walked with crutches and two long leg braces. I went to college, worked full time while I got my doctorate. When I was thirty-five I started using a manual wheelchair but switched to a power chair a year later. Four years after that I started to have severe neck, shoulder, and upper back pain. The damage had been done. I couldn't work anymore. The pain continued to get worse. I now can't dress or get in or out of the wheelchair or the bed by myself.

Childhood surgeries, walked with crutches and two long leg braces, a doctoral degree, severe upper body pain requiring a manual and then a power wheelchair—couldn't be anything but a polio survivor with PPS. Yet it turns out that Penny has spina bifida, a congenital condition in which the spinal cord doesn't finish developing and motor and sensory neurons do not form. Kids with spina bifida are often paralyzed from the waist down, different from polio survivors only in that those with spina bifida typically can't feel their legs. Spinal cord motor neurons aren't failing in those with spina bifida, because there aren't any neurons to fail. But years of walking with crutches have led to overuse-abuse of joints and muscles, causing severe chronic pain and loss of function.

Like polio survivors, kids with spina bifida were strapped into braces, given crutches, and told to walk despite severe muscle weakness or even paralysis of all leg muscles. It is finally being asked whether those born with spina bifida today are being done a disservice—now that there are laws about wheelchair accessibility—by being forced, as polio survivors were, to "walk" without leg muscles. Shouldn't kids born with spina bifida—as well as those who contract polio today wherever they are in the world—benefit from the experience of adult polio survivors who learned the hard way that "using" leads to "losing" and that preventing late-onset disability, loss of functioning, independence, and even livelihood can be prevented by conserving and preserving from childhood on?

I noticed a loss of endurance and greater fatigue after pneumonia in 1974 and they've been with me ever since. I sharply limited my social life, no longer had any physical forms of recreation, and was spending all my time either working or resting. I also developed low back pain. And there's definitely arm weakness. About once every two years I decide that I've got to have some kind of arm exercise so I do a very slow, very cautious exercise using light weights. It feels great for about three weeks. Then my arm muscles just damn well hurt and keep on burning for days; then I don't exercise anymore. Shoulder pain is clearly related to activity, and my shoulders have worn out. I switched to a van ten years ago to avoid wheelchair-to-car transfers. I switched to a power chair five years ago to avoid pushing and bought a Surehands overhead track lift to avoid wheelchair-to-bed transfers. Do I have anything left to lose?

C'mon! Loss of endurance and fatigue, low back pain, shoulder pain, and arm weakness after exercise. This has to be PPS! Well, no. Barry is paraplegic and began having these symptoms at age forty-eight, seventeen years after his spinal cord injury. It seems that no one with a long-term disability is immune from their own post-disability syndrome. Says aging and disability specialist Bonnie Moulton, who herself is experiencing the slings and arrows of aging with CP, "Those of us with an early disability need to be educated to care for ourselves as we age. But we also need support services, access to transportation and personal care assistants in our homes, and we especially need well-trained medical professionals who don't tell thirty-year-olds, 'You should expect new symptoms and a loss of function. You're just getting old.'"

Ending on an Up Note

COULD THE POLIOVIRUS CURE PPS?

Talk about a Polio Paradox. Cell biologists Andrea Bledsoe and Casey Morrow have created what they call poliovirus "replicons"—polioviruses that have been neutralized so that they can't damage neurons and have also been hollowed out. Into the replicon's hollow has been placed a gene that causes neurons to produce not poliovirus proteins, but proteins of the scientists' choosing.

Bledsoe and Morrow injected replicons into the spinal cord of mice whose neurons were specially engineered to grow poliovirus receptors. The poliovirus receptors latched on to the "Trojan horse" poliovirus replicons, which were taken inside the motor neuron—and the inserted gene went to work making a nonpoliovirus protein. The hope is that replicons will be able to get inside polio survivors' damaged brain and spinal cord neurons, insert genes for human proteins, restore failing neurons, and reverse some PPS symptoms. But there are significant hurdles to overcome.

First, you can't inject anything into a polio survivor's spinal cord or brain stem without causing more damage to the remaining, functioning neurons. Casey Morrow thinks that replicons could instead be injected into the spinal fluid, where they would get into the neurons via the poliovirus receptors as did the original poliovirus. However, I mentioned in chapter 8 that about 20 percent of polio survivors who have PPS also have antibodies to poliovirus in their spinal fluid—antibodies that might interact with and disable the replicons.

Second, if replicons do enter poliovirus-damaged neurons, what protein would they tell the neurons to produce that could repair damaged neurons? "Our goal would be to use replicons that would produce nerve growth factors, which have shown potential to induce neuron regrowth," says Morrow. "Extensive preclinical testing will be needed to determine which factor, or combination, will be effective."

Recent experiments in mice suggest that nerve growth factor protein itself might be of help. Neuroscientist Jonathan Cooper found he could increase the size of neurons by injecting NGF directly into the brains of mice. Increasing neuron size might be helpful, since remaining poliovirus-damaged motor neurons are smaller and their axons are thinner than normal. But bigger is not necessarily better. NGF would also have to repair poliovirus-damaged protein factories, which we discussed are breaking apart in polio survivors who have new muscle weakness. What's more, NGF—or whatever protein is inserted—would need to unplug the tubules within the neurons that were stopped up during the poliovirus attack. New proteins won't help much if they can't get to where they need to go.

How soon might poliovirus replicons be available to test on polio survivors with PPS? "I can't really say," says Morrow. "I do not envision the replicons initially going into polio survivors. More than likely, the replicons would be used to treat spinal cord injury causing paralysis or ALS (Lou Gehrig's disease). The pre-clinical testing on mice, and later on monkeys, would be needed to address safety issues. I would hope that within the next five or so years, new, safe therapies will be available."

Will the poliovirus itself turn out to be the cure for PPS? We'll have to wait and see. But even if the substantial hurdles can be overcome and replicons containing protein-manufacturing genes revitalize poliovirus-damaged neurons, there must be remaining neurons to be rebuilt. Even if the replicon cavalry arrives as soon as five years from now, polio survivors must save the neurons they have left by following The Golden Rule.

IS POLIO A GOOD BAD THING?

I may sound like Pollyanna, but there may actually be benefits to having gotten polio, or at least a benefit to being susceptible to it. Biology graduate student Shanda Davis surveyed polio survivors and the alumni of Drew University, asking if they had been diagnosed with Alzheimer's disease. Remarkably, 3.6 percent of the Drew alumni had Alzheimer's, but only 0.3 percent of the polio survivors did. Polio survivors had twelve times less Alzheimer's disease than those who'd never had polio. I bet you're thinking that this must be a mistake. But we went back to our own patients and found that only 0.4 percent of the polio survivors who have ever been evaluated at The Post-Polio Institute had Alzheimer's disease.

If these percentages are correct, how could having had polio protect you from getting Alzheimer's disease? Shanda Davis has a hunch. The gene that makes the poliovirus receptor is found on chromosome 19. The poliovirus receptor gene shares its DNA with a gene that makes another protein called APOE-4—a protein that is associated with getting Alzheimer's disease. You can inherit one APOE-4 gene from each parent. Those who get two APOE-4 genes have the highest risk for Alzheimer's. Those who only inherit one APOE-4 gene have a lesser risk, while those who inherit no APOE-4 genes have the lowest risk of all. Without an APOE-4 gene on chromosome 19, the poliovirus receptor gene doesn't have to share any of its DNA and may be more able to make poliovirus receptors. Without the APOE-4 you would be more likely to have more poliovirus receptors and to get polio as a child, but be less likely to make APOE-4 and to get Alzheimer's disease as an adult. Maybe even the dark cloud of polio has a silver lining.

A Millennial Medical Manifesto

Polio survivors' painful experiences during the last century provide a cautionary tale offering powerful lessons for both doctors and those with disabilities, lessons that have not yet been learned.

"The Tribal Drum"

It is still believed that people with disabilities must become "normal" because disability is not just undesirable, it is absolutely unacceptable. This belief results from "The Tribal Drum" that beats in all societies, warning members of a tribe against the danger of "the others," those who look different, who are not members of my tribe. The Tribal Drum's message results in overt abuses, from religious warfare in Northern Ireland and the Middle East to ethnic cleansing in Yugoslavia and Rwanda, neo-Nazi racial purification in Germany and America, and the ravings of Osama bin Laden. But The Drum's messages can also be subtle, permeating a society to produce covert—although no less destructive—behavior.

The Drum's most subtly destructive effect may be when negative messages about "the others" are accepted and retransmitted by the very people who supposedly have dedicated their lives to helping others. How many polio survivors, chronic fatigue and fibromyalgia patients have been discarded by doctors who thought them to be lazy or faking when an antidepressant didn't cure their fatigue, or when physical therapy on a treadmill or an exercise bicycle made weakness worse, not better?

Unfortunately, the fact that polio was not cured by the vaccine was a slap in the face to the medical establishment, and polio survivors' atrophied muscles, braces, and crutches are evidence that doctors are not gods, omniscient and omnipotent. The emergence of PPS gave a slap to the other cheek, reminding doctors of their limitations as mere mortals. In this new millennium medicine must not be about doctors' egos and their ability to "cure" disease. Medicine must become health *care,* where the goal is not curing patients with disabilities but helping them feel well and have a better quality of life.

It is also unfortunate that many of those with disabilities have had their own attitudes shaped by The Tribal Drum. Their notion of how they "should" look and act, shaped by the messages the media pounds into everyone about normalcy, certainly does not include a cane, or brace, or wheelchair. A great paradox is that those who have disabilities also listen to The Tribal Drum, adopt society's negative stereotypes, and discriminate against *themselves* because of having a disability.

It may in fact have been the polio experience, polio survivors' bodies' ability to regain function through years of painful surgeries and punishing physical therapies—as well as the polio vaccine itself—that started The Tribal Drum beating in America. The Drum's message went out across the globe: There is *no* disease that cannot be conquered by pouring money into finding a cure or a preventive vaccine; there is *no* disability that cannot be conquered if patients will only screw their courage to the sticking place, submit to surgeries, apply all their energy and the force of their own will to physical therapy—ignoring physical and emotional pain—and work hard and then harder to get "normal." It is this ethic that allows doctors to reject patients whose conditions cannot be diagnosed with a blood test or an X ray, to dismiss those who are disabled by fatigue or pain as lazy or crazy. All people with disabilities must assert themselves and stop doctors and therapists from beating The Tribal Drum. Even more, they must be vigilant to stop themselves from beating The Drum and accepting its negative messages.

Knowledge, Power, and Responsibility

The advent of the Internet has put the world's medical knowledge at everyone's fingertips. Those with disabilities—everyone with any medical diagnosis—must mine the wealth of medical information available to them and use doctors not as ultimate authorities, but as expert consultants and advisers. Patients and doctors must join in a partnership where decisions are made together, not only about how to treat a specific condition but also about how to manage its symptoms, maintain function, and maximize quality of life. We all need to embrace our new power as informed consumers, take responsibility for our own well-being, and "shop" for the most receptive, knowledgeable and compassionate medical professionals.

Unfortunately, *health care* has become an oxymoron. The experience of polio survivors during the last millennium is an example of what the health care system must no longer be. We can hope circumstances will change in the new millennium. But for polio survivors, there's no more time—or neurons—to waste! Take what you have learned in these pages, incorporate that knowledge with your life experience, accept responsibility for your own well-being, and embrace your power, as an individual and as a member of the worldwide family of polio survivors, twenty million strong. Don't let this final Polio Paradox be polio survivors' epitaph:

POLIO SURVIVORS KNEW EVERYTHING ABOUT PPS BUT DID NOTHING TO HELP THEMSELVES.

Instead, let this be polio survivors' credo:

> There is no more time to waste.
> I will listen to my body.
> I will listen to my heart.
> I will care for myself as I have cared for others.
> I will discard "normal" to ensure my ability to function
> and maintain my quality of life.
> I will thrive in spite of PPS by embracing who I am:
> A Polio *Survivor.*

May you become a new polio survivor.
May every Polio Paradox end here.

THE POST-POLIO LETTER

Basic facts about PPS for polio survivors, doctors, family & friends.

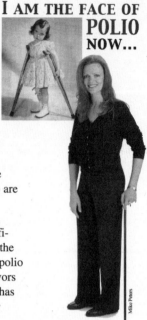

I AM THE FACE OF POLIO NOW...

Chris Templeton
Actor / Polio Survivor

Dr. Richard L. Bruno
Chairperson, International Post-Polio Task Force
Director, The Post-Polio Institute and
International Centre for Post-Polio Education and Research
Englewood (NJ) Hospital and Medical Center, USA

WHAT ARE POST-POLIO SEQUELAE? Post-Polio Sequelae (PPS, "Post-Polio Syndrome," The Late Effects of Poliomyelitis) are the unexpected and often disabling symptoms—overwhelming fatigue, muscle weakness, muscle and joint pain, sleep disorders, heightened sensitivity to anesthesia, cold and pain, as well as difficulty swallowing and breathing—that occur about 35 years after the poliovirus attack in 75% of paralytic and 40% of "nonparalytic" polio survivors. There are about 2 million North American polio survivors and 20 million polio survivors worldwide. The existence of PPS has been verified by articles in many medical journals, including *The Journal of the American Medical Association*, the *American Journal of Physical Medicine and Rehabilitation,* and *The New England Journal of Medicine*.

WHAT CAUSES PPS? PPS is caused by decades of "overuse-abuse." The poliovirus damaged 95% of brain stem and spinal cord motor neurons, killing at least 50%. Virtually every muscle in the body was affected by polio, as were brain-activating neurons that keep the brain awake and focus attention. Although damaged, the remaining neurons compensated by sending out "sprouts," like extra telephone lines, to activate muscles that were orphaned when their neurons were killed. These oversprouted, poliovirus-damaged neurons are now failing and dying from overuse, causing muscle weakness and fatigue. Overuse of weakened muscles causes muscle and joint pain, as well as difficulty with breathing and swallowing.

HOW IS PPS DIAGNOSED? There is no diagnostic test for PPS, including the electromyogram (EMG). PPS is diagnosed by excluding all other possible causes for new symptoms, including abnormal breathing and muscle twitching that commonly disturb polio survivors' sleep, a slow thyroid, and anemia. Other neurological or muscle diseases are almost never the cause of PPS symptoms.

IS PPS LIFE THREATENING? No. But because of damaged brain-activating neurons, polio survivors are extremely sensitive to—and need lower doses of—gas and intravenous anesthetics and sedative medication. Polio survivors can have difficulty waking from anesthesia and can have breathing and swallowing problems, even when given a local dental anesthetic.

IS PPS A PROGRESSIVE DISEASE? PPS is neither progressive nor a disease. PPS is caused by the body tiring of doing too much work for too long with too few poliovirus-damaged, oversprouted neurons. However, polio survivors with *untreated* muscle weakness were found to lose about 7% of their remaining, overworked motor neurons each year.

IS THERE TREATMENT FOR PPS? Yes. Polio survivors need to "conserve to preserve," conserve energy and stop overusing and abusing their bodies to preserve their abilities. Polio survivors must walk less, use needed assistive devices—braces, canes, crutches, wheelchairs—plan rest periods throughout the day, and stop activities *before* symptoms start. Also, since many polio survivors are hypoglycemic, fatigue and muscle weakness decrease when they eat protein at breakfast and small, more frequent, low-fat / higher-protein meals during the day.

ISN'T EXERCISE THE ONLY WAY TO STRENGTHEN WEAK MUSCLES? No. Muscle strengthening exercise adds to overuse. Pumping iron and "feeling the burn" means that polio-damaged neurons are burning out. Polio survivors typically can't do strenuous exercise to condition their hearts. Stretching can be helpful. But whatever the therapy, it must not trigger or increase PPS symptoms.

IS TREATMENT FOR PPS EFFECTIVE? Yes. The worst case is that PPS symptoms plateau when polio survivors stop overuse-abuse. Most polio survivors have significant decreases in fatigue, weakness, and pain once they start taking care of themselves and any sleep disorders are treated. However, because of emotionally painful past experiences related to having a disability, many polio survivors have great difficulty caring for themselves, slowing down and especially with "looking disabled" by asking for help and using assistive devices.

WHAT CAN DOCTORS, FAMILY, AND FRIENDS DO TO HELP? Polio survivors have spent their lives trying to act and look "normal." Using a brace they discarded in childhood and reducing overly full daily schedules is frightening and difficult. So friends and family need to be supportive of lifestyle changes, accept survivors' physical limitations and any new assistive devices. Most importantly, friends and family need to be willing to take on taxing physical tasks that polio survivors may be able to do but should not do. Doctors, friends, and family need to know about the cause and treatment of PPS and listen when polio survivors need to talk about how they feel about PPS and lifestyle changes. But friends and family shouldn't take control of polio survivors' lives. Neither gentle reminders nor well-meant nagging will force polio survivors to eat breakfast, use a cane, or rest between activities. Polio survivors need to be responsible for caring for their own bodies and asking for help when they need it.

Whether you had polio or not, please COPY and MAIL this letter to your doctors. With your help every doctor will learn about the cause and treatment of PPS and give polio survivors the care we so desperately need. *Thank you!*

Mia Farrow, polio survivor
Co-Chairperson, The POST-POLIO
LETTER Campaign

Thaddeus Farrow, polio survivor
Co-Chairperson, The POST-POLIO
LETTER Campaign

For more information about the cause and treatment of PPS go to www.postpolioinfo.com.

REFERENCES

More than twelve hundred books, scientific and medical journal articles, symposium discussions, personal documents, and letters were reviewed in writing *The Polio Paradox*. If they were all listed, there wouldn't be much room left for the book. So I've limited this section to only the articles mentioned and references that will best allow you, your family, doctors, and therapists to understand and treat PPS. To save more space, you'll be referred back to numbered references in previous chapters. If an author has written several articles, sometimes I'll list only the most recent publication, in which earlier papers are referenced. Articles that contain many references to other publications of interest are followed by ®. Our articles, which include references to many other publications, are available at www.postpolioinfo.com. Only the first author of an article will be given, and these abbreviations will be used:

AJPMR: *American Journal of Physical Medicine and Rehabilitation*
Am: American
APMR: *Archives of Physical Medicine and Rehabilitation*
IPC: First International Poliomyelitis Conference. Philadelphia: Lippincott, 1949.
J: Journal
LEP: *Late Effects of Poliomyelitis*. Miami: Symposia Foundation, 1985.

Med: Medicine, Medical
NYAS: *Annals of the New York Academy of Sciences,* 1995; 753
RCA: *Research and Clinical Aspects of the Late Effects of Poliomyelitis.* Birth Defects: Original articles series, 1987; 23.
Rehabil: Rehabilitation
Special PPS issues of the journal *Orthopedics:*
        ORTHO1: 1985; 8
        ORTHO2: 1991; 14
        ORTHO3: 1991; 14

Paradox. Lost.

1.   Jones D. Cardiorespiratory responses to aerobic training by patients with postpoliomyelitis sequelae. *J Am Med Association,* 1989; 261: 3255–8.
2.   Dalakas M. A long-term follow-up study of patients with post-poliomyelitis neuromuscular symptoms. *New England J Med,* 1986; 314: 959–63.

Chapter 1. In the Beginning

1.   Albom M. *Tuesdays with Morrie.* New York: Doubleday, 1997.
2.   Bruno R. Motor and sensory functioning with changing ambient temperature in post-polio subjects. LEP: 95–108.®
3.   Bruno R. Vasomotor abnormalities as post-polio sequelae. ORTHO1: 865–9.®
4.   Bruno R. Stress and "Type A" behavior as precipitants of post-polio sequelae. RCA: 145–55.®
5.   Farrow M. *What Falls Away.* New York: Nan Talese, 1997.
6.   Bruno R. Post-polio sequelae and the paradigms of the '50's: Newtie, Ozzie and Harriet versus paradigms of caring and a future for rehabilitation in America. The 45th John Stanley Coulter Memorial Lecture. APMR, 1995; 76: 1093–6.

Chapter 2. Once and Again

1.   Lane D. Late onset respiratory failure in patients with previous poliomyelitis. *Quarterly Journal Med,* 1974; 43 (172): 551–68.

2. Palmucci L. Motor neuron disease following poliomyelitis. *European Neurology*, 1980; 19: 414–18.

3. Raymond M. Paralysie essentielle de l'enfance, atrophie muscularie consecutive. *Comptes rendus de la Soc de Biology*, 1875; 27: 158.

4. Wiechers D. Late Effects of Polio: Historical perspectives. RCA: 1–11.®

Chapter 3. The Guided Missile

1. Baker AB. Neurologic signs of bulbar poliomyelitis. ICP: 241–244.

2. Barnhart M. Distribution of lesions of the brain stem in poliomyelitis. *Archives Neurology Psychiatry*, 1948; 59: 368–77.

3. Belnap D. Three-dimensional structure of poliovirus receptor bound to poliovirus. *Proceedings National Academy of Sciences USA*, 2000; 97: 73–8.

4. Bodian D. Motoneuron disease and recover in experimental poliomyelitis. LEP: 45–55.

5. Bodian D. Polioviruses. In Horsfall D (ed.): *Viral and Rickettsial Infections of Man*. Philadelphia: Lippincott, 1965.®

6. Bodian D. Histopathological basis of clinical findings in poliomyelitis. *Am J Med*, 1949; 6: 563–78.®

7. Bodian D. Poliomyelitis: Neuropathologic observations in relation to motor symptoms. *J Am Med Association*, 1947; 134: 1148–54.

8. Bodian D. Experimental nonparalytic poliomyelitis. *Bulletin Johns Hopkins Hospital*, 1945; 76: 1–17.

9. Bodian D. The pathology of early arrested and non-paralytic poliomyelitis. *Bulletin Johns Hopkins Hospital*, 1941; 69: 135–47.

10. Brown R. The bulbar form of poliomyelitis. *J Am Med Association*, 1947; 135: 425–8.

11. Bruno R. Paralytic versus "non-paralytic" polio: A distinction without a difference? AJPMR, 1999; 79: 4–12.®

12. Bruno R. Polioencephalitis and the brain fatigue generator model of post-viral fatigue syndromes. *J Chronic Fatigue Syndrome*, 1996; 2: 5–27.®

13. Bruno R. Polioencephalitis, stress and the etiology of post-polio sequelae. ORTHO2: 1269–76.®

14. Freistadt M. Correlation between poliovirus type 1 Mahoney replication in blood cells and neurovirulence. *J Virology,* 1996; 70: 6486–92.®

15. Gromeier M. Expression of the human poliovirus receptor/CD155 gene during development of the central nervous system. *Virology,* 2001; 273: 248–57.®

16. Gromeier M. Mechanism of injury-provoked poliomyelitis. *J Virology,* 1998; 72: 5056–60.®

17. Howe H. Neuropathological evidence on the portal of entry problem in human poliomyelitis. *Bulletin Johns Hopkins Hospital,* 1941: 69: 183–214.

18. Luhan J. Epidemic poliomyelitis. *Archives Pathology,* 1946; 42: 245–60.

19. Ohka S. Recent insights into poliovirus pathogenesis. *Trends in Microbiology,* 2001; 9: 501–6.

20. Matzke J. Poliomyelitis: A study of the midbrain. *Archives Neurology Psychiatry,* 1951; 65: 1–15.

21. Miller D. Human chromosome 19 carries a poliovirus receptor gene. *Cell,* 1974; 1: 167–73.

22. Miller D. Post-polio syndrome spinal cord pathology. NYAS: 186–93.

23. Morrison L. Direct spread of reovirus from the intestinal lumen to the central nervous system through vagal autonomic nerve fibers. *Proceedings National Academy of Sciences USA,* 1991; 88: 3852–6.

24. Peers J. The pathology of convalescent poliomyelitis in man. *Am J Pathology,* 1942; 19: 673–95.

25. Pezeshkpour G. Pathology of spinal cord in post-poliomyelitis muscular atrophy. RCA: 229.

26. Sabin A. Pathogenesis of poliomyelitis. *Science,* 1956: 1151–7.

27. Sharrard W. Muscle recovery in poliomyelitis. *J Bone & Joint Surgery,* 1955; 37: 63–79.

28. Shaw E. The infrequent incidence of nonparalytic poliomyelitis. *J Pediatrics,* 1954; 44: 237–43.

29. The Committee on Typing of the National Foundation for Infantile Paralysis. Immunologic classification of poliomyelitis viruses. *Am J Hygiene,* 1951; 54: 191–204.

30. Wiechers D. Reinnervation after acute poliomyelitis. RCA: 213–20.

31. Wyatt H. Poliomyelitis and infantile paralysis. History and Philosophy of Life Science, 1993; 15: 357–96.®

Chapter 4. An Awesome Thing

Chapter 3: 9, 13.

1. Aycock W. Family aggregation of polio. *West Virginia Med J,* 1934; 30–48.

2. Aycock W. The frequency of poliomyelitis in pregnancy. *New England J Med,* 1941; 225: 405–8.

3. Berg R. *Polio and Its Problems.* Philadelphia: Lippincott, 1948.

4. Bowers V. The significance of poliomyelitis during pregnancy. *Am J Obstetrics & Gynecology,* 1953; 65: 34–9.

5. Bruno R. Parallels between post-polio fatigue and chronic fatigue syndrome: A common patholophysiology? *Am J Med,* 1998; 105 (3A): 66–73.®

6. Carter H. Congenital poliomyelitis. *Obstetrics & Gynecology,* 1956; 8: 373–4.

7. Collins S. The incidence of poliomyelitis and its crippling effects as recorded in family surveys. *Public Health Reports,* 1946; 61: 327–55.

8. Dormer A. Poliomyelitis throughout the world. ICP: 348.

9. Galishoff S. Newark and the great polio epidemic of 1916. *New Jersey History,* 1976; 94: 101–11.

10. Gudnadotti M. Experience of vaccination with inactivated poliomyelitis vaccines in Iceland. *Development Biology Standards,* 1981; 47: 257–9.

11. Herndon C. A twin family study of susceptibility to poliomyelitis. *Am J Human Genetics,* 1951; 3: 17–46.

12. Horn P. Poliomyelitis in pregnancy: A twenty year report from Los Angeles. *Obstetrics & Gynecology,* 1955; 6: 121–37.

13. Melnick J. Development of neutralizing antibodies against the three types of poliomyelitis virus during an epidemic period. *Am J Hygiene,* 1953; 58: 207–22.

14. Nathanson N. Epidemiologic aspects of poliomyelitis eradication. *Review Infectious Disease,* 1984; 6: S308–12.

15. Nathanson N. The epidemiology of poliomyelitis. *Am J Epidemiology,* 1979; 110: 672–92.

16. Nielsen N. Intensive exposure as a risk factor for severe polio. *Scandinavian J Infectious Diseases*, 2001; 33: 301–5.

17. Paul J. The clinical epidemiology of poliomyelitis. *Med*, 1941; 20: 495–520.

18. Sabin A. Epidemiologic pattern of poliomyelitis in different parts of the world (and discussion). ICP: 3–33.

19. Sabin A. Paralytic consequence of poliomyelitis infection in different parts of the world and in different population groups. *Am J Public Health*, 1951; 41: 1215–30.

20. Sharrard W. The distribution of the permanent paralysis in the lower limb in poliomyelitis. *J Bone & Joint Surgery*, 1955; 37: 540–58.

21. Siegel M. Risk of paralytic and nonparalytic forms of poliomyelitis to household contacts. *J Am Med Association*, 1954; 155: 429–31.

22. Siegel M. Poliomyelitis in pregnancy. *J Pediatrics*, 1956; 49: 280–8.

23. Strebel M. Intramuscular injection within 30 days of immunization with oral poliovirus vaccine. *New England J Med*, 1995; 332: 500–6.

24. Weinstein L. The relation of sex, pregnancy and menstruation to susceptibility in poliomyelitis. *New England J Med*, 1951; 245: 54–8.

25. Weinstein L. A comparison of the clinical features of poliomyelitis in adults and children. *New England J Med*, 1952; 246: 296–302.

26. Weinstein L. Influence of age and sex on susceptibility and clinical manifestations in poliomyelitis. *New England J Med*, 1957; 257: 47–52.

27. Wyatt H. Is poliomyelitis a genetically-determined disease? I & II. *Medical Hypotheses*, 1975; 1: 23–42.®

Chapter 5. "The Pest House"

Chapter 3: 1. Chapter 4: 3.

1. Davis F. *Passage Through Crisis*. Indianapolis: Bobbs-Merrill, 1963.

2. Le Comte E. *The Long Road Back*. Boston: Beacon, 1957.

3. Mee C. *A Nearly Normal Life*. Boston: Little, Brown, 1999.

4. Robinson H. Psychiatric considerations in the adjustment of

patients with poliomyelitis. *New England J Med*, 1956; 254: 975–80.

5. Rogers N. What is scientific evidence? Sister Kenny, American doctors and polio therapy, 1940–1952. *Occas Pap Med History Australia*, 1993; 6: 245–55.

6. Woods R. *Tales from the Iron Lung and How I Got Out of It.* Philadelphia: University of Pennsylvania Press, 1994.

Chapter 6: You Can't Go Home Again

1. Davis F. *Passage Through Crisis.* Indianapolis: Bobbs-Merrill, 1963.

2. Douglas W. *Go East, Young Man.* New York: Random House, 1974.

3. Emory J. I had infantile paralysis. *Good Housekeeping.* March 1936: 133.

4. Plagemann B. *This Is Goggle.* New York: McGraw-Hill, 1955.

5. Robinson H. Psychiatric considerations in the adjustment of patients with poliomyelitis. *New England J Med*, 1956; 254: 975–80.

6. Rosenbaum S. Infantile paralysis the source of emotional problems in children. *Institute for Juvenile Research*, 1943: 12–3.

Chapter 7. Becoming "Normal"

Chapter 2: 4, 6. Chapter 3: 27.

1. Abom B. Late effects of poliomyelitis on muscular function and morphology. RCA: 223–8.

2. Agre J. Symptoms and clinical impressions of patients seen in a postpolio clinic. APMR, 1989; 70: 367–70.

3. Asper K. *The Abandoned Child Within.* New York: Fromm International Publishing, 1993.

4. Billig H. On re-innervation of paretic muscles by the use of their residual nerve supply. *J Neuropathology Experimental Neurology*, 1946; 5: 1–23.

5. Bruno R. The psychology of polio as prelude to post-polio sequelae. ORTHO2: 1185–93.®

6. Bruno R. The origins of "Type A" behavior and stress-induced symptoms in polio survivors. *Proceedings Society Behavioral Med*, 1989; 10: 85.

7. Colonna P. A study of paralytic scoliosis based on five hundred cases of poliomyelitis. *J Bone & Joint Surgery,* 1941; 23: 335–53.

8. Copellman F. Follow-up of one hundred children with poliomyelitis. *The Family,* 1944; 12: 189–96.

9. Creange S. Compliance with treatment for post-polio sequelae: Effect of Type A behavior, self-concept and loneliness. AJPMR, 1997; 76: 378–82.

10. Dunphy L. The steel cocoon. *Nursing History Review,* 2001; 9: 3–33.

11. Farbu E. Polio survivors—well educated and hard working. *J Neurology,* 2001; 248: 500–5.

12. Frick NM. Post-polio sequelae and the psychology of second disability. ORTHO1: 851–3.®

13. Lonnberg F. Late onset polio sequelae in Denmark. *Scandinavian J Rehab Med,* 1993; 28-S: 24–31.

14. Meyer E. Psychological consideration in a group of children with poliomyelitis. *J Pediatrics,* 1947; 31: 34–48.

15. Moustakas C. *Loneliness and Love.* Englewood Cliffs, NJ: Prentice Hall, 1972.

16. Rice E. The families of children with poliomyelitis. ICP: 308–13.

17. Seidenfeld M. The psychological sequelae of poliomyelitis in children. *The Nervous Child,* 1948; 7: 14–28.

18. Smith J. *Patenting the Sun.* New York: Anchor Books, 1990.

19. Thoren-Jonsson A. Ability and perceived difficulty in daily activities in people with poliomyelitis sequelae. *J Rehabil Med,* 2001; 33: 4–11.

20. Waring W. Influence of appropriate lower extremity orthotic management on ambulation, pain and fatigue in a postpolio population. APMR, 1989; 70: 371–5.

21. Young L. Reliability of a brief scale for assessment of coronary-prone behavior and standard measures of Type A behavior. *Perceptual Motor Skills,* 1982; 55: 1039–42.

Chapter 8. Polio Redux?

1. Abom B. Late effects of poliomyelitis on muscular function and morphology. RCA: 223–8.

2. Bruno R. Post-polio sequelae. ORTHO1: 884.

3. Julien J. Postpolio syndrome: poliovirus persistence is involved in the pathogenesis. *J Neurology,* 1999; 246: 472–6.®

4. Leon-Monzon M. Detection of poliovirus antibodies and poliovirus genome in patients with the post-polio syndrome. NYAS: 201–18.

5. Leparc-Goffart I. Evidence of presence of poliovirus genomic sequences in cerebrospinal fluid from patients with post-polio syndrome. *J Clinical Microbiology,* 1996; 34: 2023–26.

6. Kurent J. CSF viral antibodies: Evaluation in amyotrophic lateral sclerosis and late-onset postpoliomyelitis progressive muscular atrophy. *Archives Neurology,* 1979; 36: 269–73.

7. Melchers W. The postpolio syndrome: No evidence for poliovirus persistence. *Annals Neurology,* 1992; 32: 728–32.

8. Mulder D. Late progression of polio or *forme fruste* amyotrophic lateral sclerosis. *Mayo Clinic Proceedings,* 1972; 47: 756–61.

9. Muir P. Enterovirus infections of the central nervous system. *Intervirology,* 1997; 40: 153–66.®

10. Muir P. Evidence for persistent enterovirus infection of the central nervous system in patients with previous paralytic poliomyelitis. NYAS: 219–32.

11. Roivainen M. Twenty-one patients with strictly defined postpoliomyelitis syndrome: No poliovirus-specific IgM antibodies in the cerebrospinal fluid. *Annals Neurology,* 1994; 36: 115–6.

12. Salazar-Grueso E. Isoelectric focusing studies of serum and cerebrospinal fluid in patients with antecedent poliomyelitis. *Annals Neurology,* 1989; 26: 709–13.

13. Sharief M. Intrathecal immune response in patients with the post-polio syndrome. *New England J Med,* 1991; 325: 749–55.

Chapter 9. The Power Lifter's Lament

Chapter 1: 1, 2. Chapter 3: 9, 13, 22, 25, 27. Chapter 7: 9. Chapter 8: 1.

1. Agre J. Neuromuscular rehabilitation and electrodiagnosis. APMR, 2000; 81 (3 Supplement 1): S27–31.®

2. Agre J. Subjective recovery time after exhausting muscular activity in postpolio and control subjects. AJPMR, 1998; 77: 140–4.

3. Agre J. Strength, endurance, and work capacity after muscle strengthening exercise in postpolio subjects. APMR, 1997; 78: 681–6.

4. Agre J. Strength changes over time among polio survivors. APMR, 2000; 81: 1538–9.

5. Agre J. Low-intensity, alternate-day exercise improves muscle performance without apparent adverse effect in postpolio patients. AJPMR, 1996; 75: 50–8.

6. Agre J. A comparison of symptoms between Swedish and American post-polio individuals and assessment of lower limb strength. *Scandinavian J Rehabil Med,* 1995; 27: 183–92.

7. Beasley W. Quantitative muscle testing. APMR, 1961; 42: 398–425.

8. Bromberg M. Neurological normal patients with suspected postpoliomyelitis syndrome. APMR, 1991; 72: 493–7.

9. Bromberg M. Pattern of denervation in clinically uninvolved limbs in patients with prior poliomyelitis. *Electromyography Clinical Neurophysiology,* 1996; 36: 107–11.

10. Bruno R. Threshold electrical stimulation (TES): Dangerous or merely ineffective? *Post-Polio Sequelae Monograph Series,* 10 (1). Hackensack, NJ: Harvest Press, 2000.

11. Bruno R. Trauma and illness as precipitants of post-polio sequelae. *Post-Polio Sequelae Monograph Series,* 10 (2). Hackensack, NJ: Harvest Press, 2000.

12. Campbell M. Secondary health conditions among middle-aged individuals with chronic physical disabilities: Implications for unmet needs for services. *Assistive Technology,* 1999; 11: 105–22.

13. Campbell M. *Late Life Effects of Early Life Disability.* Downey, CA: Rancho Los Amigos Medical Center, 1993.

14. Dean E. Movement energetics of individuals with a history of poliomyelitis. APMR, 1993; 74: 478–83.®

15. Dekosky S. Elevated corticosterone levels: A possible cause of reduced axon sprouting in aged animals. *Neuroendocrinology,* 1984; 38: 33–8.

16. Dinsmore S. A double-blind, placebo-controlled trial of high-dose prednisone for the treatment of post-poliomyelitis syndrome. NYAS: 303–13.

17. Einarsson G. Muscle conditioning in late poliomyelitis. APMR, 1991; 72: 11–4.

18. Einarsson G. Muscle adaptation and disability in late poliomyelitis. *Scandinavian J Rehabil Med Supplement,* 1991; 25: 1–76.

19. Ernstoff B. Endurance training effect on individuals with poliomyelitis. APMR, 1996; 77: 843–8.

20. Feldman RM. The use of strengthening exercises in post-polio sequelae. ORTHO1: 889–90.

21. Gawne A. Post-polio syndrome. *Critical Reviews in Physical Medicine & Rehabil,* 1995; 7: 147–88.®

22. Goerss J. Fractures in an aging population of poliomyelitis survivors. *Mayo Clinic Proceedings,* 1994; 69: 333–9.

23. Grimby G. An 8-year longitudinal study of muscle strength, muscle fiber size, and dynamic electromyogram in individuals with late polio. *Muscle & Nerve,* 1998; 21: 1428–37.

24. Grimby G. Reduction in thigh muscle cross-sectional area and strength in a 4-year follow-up in late polio. APMR, 1996; 77: 1044–8.

25. Herndon C. A twin family study of susceptibility to poliomyelitis. *Am J Human Genetics,* 1951; 3: 17–46.

26. Ivanyi B. Muscle strength in postpolio patients. *Muscle & Nerve,* 1996; 19: 738–42.

27. Ivanyi B. Macro EMG follow-up study in post-poliomyelitis patients. *J Neurology,* 1994; 242: 37–40.

28. Kerezoudi E. Influence of age on regeneration in the peripheral nervous system. *Gerontology,* 1999; 45: 301–6.

29. Klein M. Changes in strength over time among polio survivors. APMR, 2000; 81: 1059–64.

30. Klein M. The relation between lower extremity strength and shoulder overuse symptoms. APMR, 2000; 81: 789–95.

31. Klingman J. Functional recovery: A major risk factor for the development of postpoliomyelitis muscular atrophy. *Archives Neurology,* 1988; 45: 645–7.

32. Kriz J. Cardiorespiratory responses to upper extremity aerobic training by postpolio subjects. APMR, 1992; 73: 49–54.

33. Lewis C (ed.) *Orthopedic Assessment and Treatment of the Geriatric Patient.* St. Louis: C. V. Mosby, 1993.®

34. Luciano C. Reinnervation in clinically unaffected muscles of patients with prior paralytic poliomyelitis. NYAS: 394–6.

35. Mann D. Nerve cell protein metabolism and degenerative

disease. *Neuropathology & Applied Neurobiology*, 1982; 8: 161–76.

36. McComas A. Motoneurone Disease and Ageing. *Lancet*, 1973; ii: 1477–80.

37. McComas A. Early and late losses of motor units after poliomyelitis. *Brain*, 1997; 120: 1415–21.

38. Moskowitz E. Follow-up study in seventy-five cases of non-paralytic poliomyelitis. *J Am Med Association*, 1953; 152: 1505–6.

39. Nee L. Post-polio syndrome in twins and their siblings. NYAS: 378–80.

40. Nollet F. Disability and functional assessment in former polio patients with and without postpolio syndrome. APMR, 1999; 80: 136–43.

41. Pare W. The effect of chronic environmental stress on premature aging in the rat. *J Gerontology*, 1965; 20: 78–84.

42. Peach P. Effect of treatment and non-compliance on post-polio sequelae. ORTHO2: 1199–203.

43. Perry J. Polio: Long-term problems. ORTHO1: 877–81.

44. Perry J. Findings in post-poliomyelitis syndrome: Weakness of muscles of the calf as a source of late pain and fatigue of muscles of the thigh after poliomyelitis. *J Bone & Joint Surgery*, 1995; 77: 1148–53.

45. Pitha J. Protein synthesis during aging of human cells in culture. *Experimental Cell Research*, 1975; 94: 310–4.

46. Ramlow J. Epidemiology of the post-polio syndrome. *Am J. Epidemiology*, 1992; 136: 769–86.

47. Rodriguez A. Electromyographic and neuromuscular variables in post-polio subjects. APMR, 1995; 76: 989–93.

48. Rosenheimer J. Effects of chronic stress and exercise on age-related changes in end-plate architecture. *J Neurophysiology*, 1985; 53: 1582–9.

49. Sabin A. Nature of non-paralytic and transitory paralytic poliomyelitis in rhesus monkeys inoculated with human virus. *J Experimental Med*, 1941; 73: 757–70.

50. Shaw E. The infrequent incidence of nonparalytic poliomyelitis. *J Pediatrics*, 1954; 44: 237–43.

51. Spector S. Strength gains without muscle injury after strength training in patients with postpolio muscular atrophy. *Muscle & Nerve*, 1996; 19: 1282–90.

52. Stalberg E. Dynamic electromyography and muscle biopsy changes in a 4-year follow-up study of patients with a history of polio. *Muscle & Nerve*, 1995; 18: 699–707.

53. Tollback A. Isokinetic strength, macro EMG and muscle biopsy of paretic foot dorsiflexors in chronic neurogenic paresis. *Scandinavian J Rehabil Med*, 1993; 25: 183–7.

54. Trojan D. Serum insulin-like growth factor-I (IGF-I) does not correlate positively with isometric strength, fatigue, and quality of life in post-polio syndrome. *J Neurological Science*, 2001; 182: 107–15.

55. Trojan D. A multicenter, randomized, double-blinded trial of pyridostigmine in postpolio syndrome. *Neurology*, 1999; 53: 1225–33.

56. Trojan D. Electrophysiology and electrodiagnosis of the post-polio motor unit. ORTHO3: 1353–61.

57. Shetty K. Studies of growth hormone/insulin-like growth factor-I in polio survivors. NYAS: 276–84.®

58. Stein D. A double-blind, placebo-controlled trial of amantadine for the treatment of fatigue in patients with the post-polio syndrome. NYAS: 296–302.

59. Werner R. Risk factors for median mononeuropathy of the wrist in postpoliomyelitis patients. APMR, 1989; 70: 464–7.

60. Willen C. Dynamic water exercise in individuals with late poliomyelitis. APMR, 2001; 82: 66–72.

61. Willen C. Physical performance in individuals with late effects of polio. *Scandinavian J Rehabil Med*, 1999; 31: 244–9.

62. Willen C. Pain, physical activity and disability in individuals with late effects of polio. APMR, 1998; 79: 915–9.

63. Willen C. Endurance training effect on individuals with postpoliomyelitis. APMR, 1996; 77: 843–8.

Chapter 10. Pain and the Post-Polio Brain

Chapter 2: 2, 3. Chapter 3: 6. Chapter 7: 7. Chapter 9: 30, 44, 60, 63.

1. Bodian D. Poliomyelitis: Pathologic anatomy. ICP: 62–84 (discussion: 96–105).

2. Bruno R. Preventing complications in polio survivors undergoing surgery and other procedures requiring anesthesia. *Post-Polio*

Sequelae Monograph Series, 11 (1). Hackensack, NJ: Harvest Press, 2001.

3. Colonna P. A study of paralytic scoliosis based on five hundred cases of poliomyelitis. *J Bone & Joint Surgery,* 1941; 23: 335–53.

4. Vallbona C. Response of pain to static magnetic fields in post-polio patients. APMR, 1997; 78: 1200–3.

Chapter 11. Brain Brownout

Chapter 2: 4. Chapter 3: 2, 7, 10, 12, 13, 18, 20, 24. Chapter 7: 14. Chapter 10: 2.

1. Bruno R. Word finding difficulty as a post-polio sequelae. AJPMR, 2000; 79: 343–8.®

2. Bruno R. Elevated plasma prolactin and EEG slow wave power in post-polio fatigue. *J Chronic Fatigue Syndrome,* 1998; 4: 61–76.®

3. Bruno R. Bromocriptine in the treatment of post-polio fatigue. AJPMR, 1996; 75: 340–7.

4. Bruno R. The pathophysiology of a central cause of post-polio fatigue. NYAS: 257–75.®

5. Bruno R. The neuroanatomy of post-polio fatigue. APMR, 1994; 75: 498–504.®

6. Bruno R. The neuropsychology of post-polio fatigue. APMR, 1993; 74: 1061–5.

7. Freidenberg D. Post-poliomyelitis syndrome: Assessment of behavioral features. *Neuropsychiatry, Neuropsychology & Behavioral Neurology,* 1989; 2: 272–81.

8. Holmgren B. Electro-encephalography in poliomyelitis. ICP: 448–50.

9. Magoun H. Bulbar poliomyelitis (discussion). ICP: 250.

10. Mann D. Nerve cell protein metabolism and degenerative disease. *Neuropathology & Applied Neurobiology,* 1982; 8: 161–76.

11. Pitha J. Protein synthesis during aging of human cells in culture. *Experimental Cell Research,*1975; 94: 310–4.

12. Roelcke U. Reduced glucose metabolism in the frontal cortex and basal ganglia of multiple sclerosis patients with fatigue. *Neurology,*1997; 48: 1566–71.

13. Shaw E. Bulbar poliomyelitis (discussion). ICP: 254.

14. Siddiqi Z. Age-related neuronal loss from the substantia nigra-pars compacta and ventral tegmental area of the rhesus monkey. *J Neuropathology & Experimental Neurology,* 1999; 58: 959–71.

15. Volkow ND. Association between age-related decline in brain dopamine activity and impairment in frontal and cingulate metabolism. *Am J Psychiatry,* 2000; 157: 75–80.

Chapter 12. To Sleep, Perchance to Sleep?

Chapter 2: 4. Chapter 3: 1. Chapter 10: 2.

1. Bach J. Pulmonary dysfunction and sleep disordered breathing as post-polio sequelae. ORTHO3: 1329–37.

2. Bruno R. Abnormal movements in sleep as a post-polio sequelae. AJPMR, 1998; 77: 339–43.®

3. Bruno R. Nocturnal generalized myoclonus as a post-polio sequelae. APMR, 1995; 76: 594.

4. Caldwell JA. The impact of fatigue in air medical and other types of operations: a review of fatigue facts and potential counter-measures. *Air Med J,* Jan-Feb 2001; 20: 25-32.

5. Dean A. Sleep apnea in patients with postpolio syndrome. *Annals Neurology,* 1998; 43: 661–664.

6. Fischer D. Sleep-disordered breathing as a late effect of poliomyelitis. RCA: 115–20.

7. Hsu A. Postpolio sequelae and sleep-related disordered breathing. *Mayo Clinic Proceedings,* 1998; 73: 216–24.

8. Lin M. Pulmonary function and spinal characteristics: Their relationships in persons with idiopathic and postpoliomyelitic scoliosis. APMR, 2001; 82: 335–41.

9. Lue F. Sleep and symptoms in post polio survivors, fibromyalgia and controls. Presentation, Associated Professional Sleep Societies: 1996.

10. Robinson L. New laryngeal muscle weakness in post-polio syndrome. *Laryngoscope,* 1998; 108: 732–4.

11. Siegel H. Physiologic events initiating REM sleep in patients with the postpolio syndrome. *Neurology,* 1999; 52: 516–22.

12. Tachibana N. Sleep problems in multiple sclerosis. *European Neurology,* 1994; 34: 320–3.

13. Tamaki M. Restorative effects of a short afternoon nap (< 30 min) in the elderly on subjective mood, performance and EEG activity. *Sleep Res Online,* 2000; 3: 131-9.

Chapter 13. Baby, It's Cold Inside

Chapter 2: 2, 3. Chapter 9: 13, 34, 60. Chapter 10: 2.

1. Abramson D. Blood flow in the extremities affected by anterior poliomyelitis. *Archives Internal Med*, 1943; 71: 391–6.

2. Kottke F. Studies on increased vasomotor tone in the lower extremities following anterior poliomyelitis. APMR, 1951; 32: 401–7.

3. Smith E. Role of the sympathetic nervous system in acute poliomyelitis. *J Pediatrics*, 1949; 34: 1–11.

4. Stenport L. Treatment of cold feet and legs after poliomyelitis. *Angiology*, 1951; 2: 345–9.

5. Trott A. Peripheral circulatory changes in patients with poliomyelitis. *Clinical Orthopedics*, 1968; 61: 213–22.

Chapter 14. Blood Sugar, Blood Pressure, and the Post-Polio Belly

Chapter 2: 4. Chapter 3: 2, 7, 10, 12, 13, 18, 20, 24. Chapter 9: 6, 37. Chapter 10: 2. Chapter 12: 1.

1. Agre J. A comparison of symptoms between Swedish and American post-polio individuals and assessment of lower limb strength. *Scandinavian J Rehabil Med*, 1995; 27: 183–92.

2. Benini L. Achalasia: A possible late cause of postpolio dysphagia. *Digestive Diseases Science*, 1996: 41: 516–8.

3. Bou-Holaigah I. Provocation of hypotension and pain during upright tilt table testing in adults with fibromyalgia. *Clinical & Experimental Rheumatology*, 1997; 15: 239–46.

4. Bruno R. Preventing complications in polio survivors undergoing dental procedures. *Post-Polio Sequelae Monograph Series*, 6 (2). Hackensack, NJ: Harvest Press, 1996.

5. Bruno R. Chronic fatigue, fainting and autonomic dysfunction: Further similarities between post-polio fatigue and chronic fatigue syndrome? *J Chronic Fatigue Syndrome*, 1997; 3: 107–17.

6. Bruno R. Parasympathetic abnormalities as post-polio sequelae. APMR, 1995; 76: 594.

7. Bucholz D. Postpolio dysphagia. *Dysphagia*, 1994; 9: 99–100.®

8. Bucholz D. Post-polio dysphagia: alarm or caution?

ORTHO3: 1303–5.®

9. Calkins H. Relationship between chronic fatigue syndrome and neurally mediated hypotension. *Cardiology Review,* 1998; 6: 125–34.

10. Dantas R. Achalasia occurring years after acute polio-myelitis. *Arq Gastroenterology,* 1993; 30: 58–61.

11. Deary I. Effects of hypoglycaemia on cognitive function. In Frier B, Fisher B (eds.): *Hypoglycaemia and Diabetes.* Boston: Edward Arnold, 1993.

12. Dowhaniuk M. Dysphagia in individuals with no history of bulbar polio. NYAS: 405–7.

13. Farb A. Swallow syncope. *Maryland Med J,* 1999; 48: 151–4.

14. Gold A. The effect of I.Q. on the degree of cognitive deterioration experienced during acute hypoglycemia in normal humans. *Intelligence,* 1995; 20: 267–90.®

15. Gold A. Cognitive function during insulin-induced hypoglycemia in humans. *Psychopharmacology,* 1995; 119: 325–33.

16. Ivanyi B. Dysphagia in postpolio patients. *Dysphagia,* 1994; 9: 96–8.

17. Jacob R. Brainstem dysfunction is provoked by a less pronounced hypoglycemic stimulus in diabetic bb rats. *Diabetes,* 1995; 44: 900–5.

18. Jardine D. Baroreceptor denervation presenting as part of a vagalmononeuropathy. *Clinical Autonomic Research,* 2000; 10: 69–75.

19. Low P. Comparison of the postural tachycardia syndrome (POTS) with orthostatic hypotension due to autonomic failure. *J Autonomic Nervous System,* 1994; 50: 181–8.

20. Mahgoub A. Weakness, daytime somnolence, cough, and respiratory distress in a 77-year-old man with a history of childhood polio. *Chest,* 2001; 120: 659–61.

21. Manyari D. Abnormal reflex venous function in patients with neurally mediated syncope. *J Am College Cardiology,* 1996; 27: 1730–5.

22. McCall A. Immunohistochemical localization of the neuron-specific glucose transporter (GLUT3) to neuropil in adult rat brain. *Brain Research,* 1994; 659: 292–7.

23. Mehta D. Recurrent paroxysmal complete heart block induced by vomiting. *Chest,* 1988; 94: 433–5.

24. Palmer E. The upper gastrointestinal vagovagal reflexes that affect the heart. *Am J Gastroenterology,* 1976; 66: 513–22.

25. Ulfberg J. Sleep apnea syndrome among poliomyelitis survivors. *Neurology,* 1997; 49: 1189–90.

26. Rubin A. Near-drowning scuba diving: an unusual late sequel of bulbar polio. *J Laryngology & Otolaryngology,* 1984; 98: 733–6.

27. Schondorf R. Idiopathic postural orthostatic tachycardia syndrome. *Neurology,* 1993; 43: 132–7.

28. Silver J. Polio survivors: Falls and subsequent injuries. AJPMR, 2002 (in press).

29. Sra J. Sinus tachycardia with atrioventricular block. *J Cardiovascular Electrophysiology,* 1998; 9: 203–7.

30. Taylor L. The effects of blood sugar level changes on cognitive function, affective state and somatic symptoms. *J Behavioral Medicine,* 1988; 11: 279–91.

31. Wolkowitz O. Cognitive effects of corticosteroids. *Am J Psychiatry,* 1990; 147: 1297–303.

Chapter 15. Mind Over Matter

Chapter 2: 4. Chapter 3: 13. Chapter 7: 2, 5, 9, 19, 20. Chapter 9: 43.

1.   Bruno R. Five year follow-up to the 1985 National Post-Polio Survey. APMR, 1990; 10: 886.

2.   Creange S. Family support as a predictor of participation in rehabilitation for post-polio sequelae. *New Jersey Rehab,* 1994; 8: 8–11.

3.   Frankenhauser M. Dissociation between sympathetic-adrenal and pituitary-adrenal responses to an achievement situation characterized by high controllability: Comparison between type A and type B males and females. *Biological Psychology,* 1980; 10: 79–91.

4.   Kemp B. Depression and life satisfaction in aging polio survivors versus age-matched controls. APMR, 1997; 78: 187–92.

5.   Schanke A. Psychological distress, social support and coping behavior among polio survivors. *Disability & Rehabilitation,* 1997; 19: 108–16.

6.   Tate D. Coping with the late effects: Differences between

depressed and nondepressed polio survivors. AJPMR, 1994; 73: 27–35.

7.   Westbrook M. Living with the late effects of disability: A five year follow-up survey of coping among post-polio survivors. *Australian Occupational Therapy J*, 1996; 43: 60–71.

8.   Westbrook M. A survey of post polio sequelae. *Australian J Physiotherapy*, 199; 37: 89–102.

9.   Westbrook M. Coping with a second disability: Implications of the late effects of poliomyelitis for occupational therapists. *Australian Occupational Therapy J*, 1991; 38: 83–91.

10. Van Schijndel M. Effects of behavioral control and Type A behavior on cardiovascular responses. *Psychophysiology*, 1984; 21: 501–9.

Chapter 16. Less Is More: Managing PPS

Chapter 9: 29, 43. Chapter 15: 1.

1.   Agre J. Intermittent isometric activity: Its effect on muscle fatigue in postpolio subjects. APMR, 1991; 72: 971–5.

Chapter 17. Fatigue By Any Other Name

Chapter 3: 11, 13. Chapter 4: 5. Chapter 14: 4, 8.

1.   Adler G. Reduced hypothalamic-pituitary and sympathoad-renal responses to hypoglycemia in women with fibromyalgia syndrome. *Am J Med*, 1999; 106: 534–43.

2.   Bazelmans E. Is physical deconditioning a perpetuating factor in chronic fatigue syndrome? *Psychological Med*, 2001; 31, 107–14.

3.   Berg A. Established fibromyalgia syndrome and parvovirus B19 infection. *J Rheumatology*, 1993; 20: 194–203.

4.   Bruno R. Behavioral rehabilitation of CFS. In John J, Oleske J (eds.): *Consensus Manual for the Management of Chronic Fatigue Syndrome*. Trenton: New Jersey Academy of Medicine, 2001.

5.   Bruno R. Cincinnati's stealth polio epidemic. *New Mobility*, 1999; 10: 37–9.

6.   Cohen H. Abnormal sympathovagal balance in men with fibromyalgia. *J Rheumatology*, 2001; 28: 581–9.

7.   Dowsett E. Long term sickness absence due to ME/CFS in

UK schools. *J Chronic Fatigue Syndrome*, 1997; 3: 29–42.

8. Fuentes K. Intraindividual variability in cognitive performance in persons with chronic fatigue syndrome. *Clinical Neuropsychology*, 2001; 15: 210–27.

9. Glass J.D. Poliomyelitis due to West Nile Virus. *New England J Med*, 2002.

10. Haley R. Brain abnormalities in Gulf War syndrome. *Radiology*, 2000; 215: 807–17.

11. Haley R. Effect of basal ganglia injury on central dopamine activity in Gulf War syndrome. *Archives Neurology*, 2000; 57: 1280–5.

12. Hallegua D. Prevalence of fibromyalgia in growth hormone deficient adults. *J Musculoskeletal Pain*, 2001; 9: 35–42.

13. Huang C. A community-based study of chronic fatigue syndrome. *Archives Internal Med*, 1999; 159: 2129–37.

14. Le Bon O. How significant are primary sleep disorders and sleepiness in the chronic fatigue syndrome? *Sleep Research Online*, 2000; 3: 43–8.

15. Landis C. Decreased nocturnal levels of prolactin and growth hormone in women with fibromyalgia. *J Clinical Endocrinology Metabolism*, 2001; 86: 1672–8.

16. Laine M. Prolonged arthritis associated with sindbis-related (Pogosta) virus infection. *Rheumatology* (Oxford), 2000; 39: 1272–4.

17. Lane R. Chronic fatigue syndrome. *J Neurology, Neurosurgery & Psychiatry*, 2000; 69: 289.

18. Lange G. Brain MRI abnormalities exist in a subset of patients with chronic fatigue syndrome. *J Neurological Science*, 1999; 171: 3–7.

19. Lapp C. Exercise limits in chronic fatigue syndrome. *Am J Med*, 1997; 103: 83–4.

20. Lewis S. Psychosocial factors and chronic fatigue syndrome. *Psychological Med*, 1994; 24: 661–71.

21. McGarry F. Enterovirus in the chronic fatigue syndrome. *Annals Internal Med*, 1994; 120: 972–3.

22. Naschitz J. Cardiovascular response to upright tilt in fibromyalgia differs from that in chronic fatigue syndrome. *J Rheumatology*, 2001; 28: 1356–60.

23. Nash P. Chronic Coxsackie B infection mimicking primary

fibromyalgia. *J Rheumatology,* 1989; 16: 1506–8.

24. Pillemer S. The neuroscience and endocrinology of fibromyalgia. *Arthritis & Rheumatology,* 1997; 40: 1928–39.

25. Qiao Z. Electrodermal and microcirculatory activity in patients with fibromyalgia during baseline, acoustic stimulation and cold pressor tests. *J Rheumatology,* 1991; 18: 1383–9.

26. Richardson J. Relationship between SPECT scans and buspirone tests in patients with ME/CFS. *J Chronic Fatigue Syndrome,* 1998; 4: 23–33.®

27. Rowe P. Orthostatic intolerance and chronic fatigue syndrome associated with Ehlers-Danlos syndrome. *J Pediatrics,* 1999; 135: 494–9.

28. Sampson B.A. West Nile encephalitis: the neuro-pathology of four fatalities. *Annals NY Academy of Sciences,* 2001; 951: 172-8.

29. Shepherd C. Pacing and exercise in chronic fatigue syndrome. *Physiotherapy,* 2001; 87: 395–6.

30. Tayag-Kier C. Sleep and periodic limb movement in sleep in juvenile fibromyalgia. *Pediatrics,* 2000; 106: E70.

31. Staud R. Abnormal sensitization and temporal summation of second pain (wind-up) in patients with fibromyalgia syndrome. *Pain,* 2001; 91: 165–75.

32. Streeten DH. Role of impaired lower-limb venous innervation in the pathogenesis of the chronic fatigue syndrome. *Am J Med Science,* 2001; 321: 163–7.

33. Trojan D. Fibromyalgia is common in a postpoliomyelitis clinic. *Archives Neurology,* 1995; 52: 620–4.

34. Vaeroy H. Altered sympathetic nervous system response in patients with fibromyalgia. *J Rheumatology,* 1989; 16: 1460–5.

35. Van Houdenhove B. Pemorbid "overactive" lifestyle in chronic fatigue syndrome and fibromyalgia. *Journal of Psychosomatic Research,* 2001; 51: 571–6.®

36. White P. Graded exercise therapy for chronic fatigue syndrome. *Physiotherapy,* 2001; 87: 285–8.

37. Wittrup I. Comparison of viral antibodies in 2 groups of patients with fibromyalgia. *J Rheumatology,* 2001; 28: 601–3.

Chapter 18. No More Time to Waste

Chapter 9: 12, 13, 33.

1. Balandin S. Adults with cerebral palsy. *J Intellectual & Developmental Disability*, 1997; 22: 104–24.

2. Bledsoe A. Cytokine production in motor neurons by poliovirus replicon vector gene delivery. *Nature Biotechnology*, 2000; 18: 964–9.

3. Bruno R. "Beating" the tribal drum: Rejecting disability stereotypes and preventing self-discrimination. *Disability & Society*, 1999; 14: 855–7.

4. Dunne K. The Adult Spina Bifida Network Survey. *Insights*, 1986; 14: 28–32.

5. Machemer R. *Aging and Developmental Disabilities*. Rochester, NY: University of Rochester, 1993.

6. Moulton B. Post-everything syndrome. *New Mobility*, 2000; 9: 41–5.®

7. Segalman R. *A Personal Experience with Cerebral Palsy with Total Body Involvement: Solving Medical Problems in Midlife*. Oakland, CA: United Cerebral Palsy, 1993.

About the Author

Richard L. Bruno, H.D., Ph.D., is a clinical psychophysiologist specializing in the treatment of chronic conditions—fatigue, pain, and stress—as well as Post-Polio Sequelae (PPS). He is chairperson of The International Post-Polio Task Force, an associate professor at New York's Mount Sinai School of Medicine, and director of The Post-Polio Institute, The International Centre for Post-Polio Education and Research, and the Fatigue Management Programs at New Jersey's Englewood Hospital and Medical Center. Bruno is internationally recognized as the world's foremost expert on PPS. Dr. Bruno received an honorary Doctor of Humanics degree from Springfield College in 1998.